Topics in Down Syndrome

Third Edition

Fine Motor Skills for Children with Down Syndrome

A Guide for Parents and Professionals

Maryanne Bruni, BScOT (Reg)

D1260433

Woodbine House

Text © 2006, 2016 Maryanne Bruni
Illustrations on pages 258-76 © Sue Yurkewich

All rights reserved under International and Pan-American copyright conventions. Published in the United States of America by Woodbine House, Inc., 6510 Bells Mill Rd., Bethesda, MD 20817. 800-843-7323.

Library of Congress Cataloging-in-Publication Data

Bruni, Maryanne.
  Fine motor skills for children with Down syndrome : a guide for parents and professionals / Maryanne Bruni. -- Third edition.
     pages cm
  Includes bibliographical references and index.
  ISBN 978-1-60613-259-3 (pbk.)
  1. Down syndrome. 2. Motor learning. 3. Motor ability in children. I. Title.
  RJ506.D68B78 2015
  618.92'858842--dc23

                                                                            2015032140

Manufactured in the United States of America

10 9   8   7   6   5   4   3

Fine Motor Skills for Children with Down Syndrome

To my parents, Andrew and Mary Burghardt,
and to my in-laws, Pasquale and Gina Bruni

Table of Contents

Acknowledgements

My sincere thanks go out to all those who have helped me personally and professionally in the writing of this book. Thank you to:

- All the persons who have Down syndrome that I have had the privilege to meet over the years, many of whom I have watched grow up into fine young men and women. Your refreshing approach to life helps me stay focused on what is important.
- All the families of children with Down syndrome I have had the privilege of knowing over the years. Your commitment to your sons, daughters, brothers, sisters, etc. is an inspiration. Thank you to all the families who agreed to the use of photos of their children in this book.
- The professional colleagues I have worked with and consulted with, who shared generously their time and expertise.
- The Director of Silver Creek Pre-School, Susan Slezak Kawa, and all the dedicated therapists and teachers I have worked with there over many years. Many children who have Down syndrome have attended Silver Creek Pre-School in Toronto; they and their families have found support and expertise at Silver Creek.
- The Canadian Occupational Therapy Foundation for their publication grant, which gave me the financial and professional support to complete the first edition of the book.
- All the families in Canada and the United States who filled out the Sensory Profile and Sensory Questionnaire, and to Dr. Debra Mosnyk Cameron, PhD OT (Reg), Shelly Dua, MScOT, and Sarah Noy, MScOT, who worked with me on the research into reported

sensory processing in children with Down syndrome, which helped inform the chapter on Sensory Processing.

- Susan Stokes, editor at Woodbine House, simply the best possible editor to work with, and to her team at Woodbine House.
- Sue Yurkewich for her work on the pencil control worksheet graphics.
- My daughters, Meghan, Alison, and Sarah, who have provided me with the rewarding perspective of the continuum of development as they have grown into adulthood, and whose commitment to the dignity of all persons is inspiring to all.
- My husband, Romeo, who is always there with love and encouragement, and whose dedication to providing medical care to all persons in their homes is unrelenting.

Introduction:
A Parent's Perspective

Twenty-six years ago our family began a new journey. We had already embarked on the journey of parenthood, having been blessed with two daughters already. When Sarah was born with Down syndrome, it added a new dimension to our lives as a family. In some ways it was like taking a trip without a map—with detours along the way, not really knowing if we were headed in the right direction. It has also been a journey with unexpected rewards, and has helped define life directions for each member of our family.

I have had a thirty-six-year career as an occupational therapist. Although I had worked with children with special needs prior to Sarah's birth, my experience with children with Down syndrome was limited. As parents of a child with Down syndrome, we had to navigate the emotional roadmap and learn to become knowledgeable advocates for Sarah, just as all other families do.

My professional training and experience gave me a framework with which to observe and understand the stages of Sarah's development. By her responses, Sarah helped me recognize learning and developmental opportunities that are motivating, realistic, and practical. Through the day-to-day reality of raising her, I became more aware of how small changes to an activity or task can make a significant difference between success and failure, motivation and frustration. I learned how to provide opportunities for Sarah's development and practice of skills through the many daily activities in our home.

Development for our children with Down syndrome unfolds according to each child's own internal schedule, as it does for all children. It is usually slower to unfold, and our children benefit from help along the way. As parents and professionals, we need ideas that are practical, are easy to carry out, can be used spontaneously, and are motivating and fun for our children. So many aspects of our children's development may need help that it can be overwhelming at times for parents.

All children have their own internal strengths and limitations, and sometimes, no matter how dedicated and committed you are as a parent, your child may not be able to learn a particular skill at that particular time. Rather than struggle, I learned to let it go and move on to something else, and often the challenging skill emerged when Sarah was ready. In my personal and professional experience, many children (including those with Down syndrome) are tuned in to the underlying agenda of adults and to the emotional climate of the situation.

Each stage of life presents new challenges and new opportunities for growth. As Sarah grew and her needs evolved, so the focus of our attention to support her evolved. With each passing year, Sarah's world widened and so did the scope of our network and advocacy. Perspectives and expectations change as our children enter adulthood. The years of input from developmental specialists and therapists are largely behind us. Sarah is now an adult, twenty-six years old, and has established her own life preferences and priorities. She continues to add skills, abilities, and interests as an adult. As I had hoped, Sarah's fine motor skills have contributed to her ability to manage many aspects of her life as an adult. I recognize that all the small steps, the little achievements, and experiences she has had have ultimately given Sarah a feeling of self-worth that will continue to guide her through her life.

All parents want the best for their child. Providing a safe, loving home environment that meets the physical, emotional and safety needs of our child are our primary concerns. By actively recognizing and validating the inherent dignity of our children as valued persons in our communities, we help foster a mindset of inclusion and possibility.

How to Use This Book

In this book I will share my experience and current best practices about sensory processing and the development of fine motor skills in children, teens and adults with Down syndrome through daily home, school, work, and community activities. My intent is that this book will be of use to parents, teachers, and health professionals.

I present a visual model of how hand skills develop, represented by the building of a house. This is explained in Chapter 1, and will help you understand how motor development prepares your child to be able to do "fine motor skills" such as holding and using a pencil. Chapter 2 focuses on the steps in learning, how to take things one step at a time, and thoughts on motivating your child. Most of the activities in this book can be done at home or school, without special equipment, using materials that are readily available. Chapter 3 discusses the physical and medical characteristics of Down syndrome that can affect fine motor skill development. An outline of the kinds of skills that will be emerging at different ages is presented. Chapter 4 explains fine motor development in infancy, as it relates to gross motor milestones. Ideas for positioning and play activities to prepare your baby for fine motor skill development are presented.

Chapters 5, 6, and 7 explain the foundation skills for fine motor abilities. These foundations, called stability, bilateral coordination, and sensation, are like the building blocks upon which children can develop the precise movements of their hands. The foundation skills develop throughout childhood, and are relevant for all ages. Chapter 8 begins to describe and give ideas for dexterity, which is really what we think of as "fine motor skills." You will read about how your child learns to pick up and let go of things, and develops coordinated hand movements. This chapter is particularly relevant for the toddler and preschooler who is developing patterns of grasping and release during play.

Chapter 9 carries the discussion into school-related tasks, such as printing, cutting, and the use of computers and technology. The normal development of pencil grasp is described, and activities to promote visual motor skills are suggested. Parents of preschoolers, school-aged children, and teens will find this chapter relevant. A special feature called "Grandma's and Grandpa's List" is included at the ends of Chapters 4 through 11. This is a list of suggested toys and activities that will help your child's development in each area. It may help you come up with ideas if interested friends and relatives ask you what gifts to buy for your child for birthdays and holidays.

Chapter 10 covers self-help skills (dressing, eating and drinking, and grooming). Practical suggestions for adaptations and ideas for common dressing problems are outlined. Household chores and leisure activities are also relevant to fine motor development, and they are briefly explored in this chapter. These activities become increasingly important as children with Down syndrome mature into adolescence and adulthood. Independent living and work skills are also briefly discussed in this chapter. Young men and women with Down syndrome who have developed and practiced the fine motor abilities needed for self-help as children can spend their energies as adults on organizing their time and taking responsibility for managing their daily living skills as independently as possible.

Chapter 11 provides an overview of sensory processing. Some of the ways that sensory processing can affect behavior, fine motor development, and the development of self-help skills are discussed. Strategies to assist parents in helping their child deal with sensory processing issues are presented. Sensory processing is important, as it can not only affect motor development, but also the emotional state of the child, and ability to focus and maintain attention, which, in turn, affects his ability to learn new skills.

In this book, I have made a point of suggesting activities that can be incorporated into daily routines and play time. I know how hard it is as a parent to find the time to sit down and do "therapy" or "teaching" with your child, especially when the child perceives it as such. There is definitely a need and place for doing structured teaching and therapy, and our children benefit from it. However, if we interact with our children only in a structured format, and take on the role of a teacher or therapist much of the time, we may end up frustrated, and our child resistant.

When you read through this book, you will probably recognize some activities that may interest your child and others that won't. Choose a few that you think will be of interest; that your child will be able to do without too much difficulty. Then think about how you can incorporate them into your daily routines, so that you do not always have to set aside extra time to do them with your child.

In this book, I have described the *components* of fine motor development rather than *stages* of development. I did this because, at any stage of development, several components of fine motor skills (types of movement and control) are developing at once. To give a sense of the continuity of development of each type of skill, I chose to present each skill individually. Throughout the book, particularly in Chapter 3, there are references to how all the separate skills come together. A child of any age will be developing the various components of fine motor skills simultaneously. Therefore, parents may find it useful to choose activities from more than one chapter at once.

A Model of Hand Skill Development

The development of a child is a wondrous thing, involving a series of seemingly miraculous unfoldings of personality, emotions, relationships, and movements. And it is no less wondrous when the unfoldings occur more slowly, as for our children with Down syndrome. In fact, the achievement of every milestone and development can be the cause for celebration in many families. When Sarah learned to articulate a new sound as a child, or did her buttons up for the first time, or did anything at all that was a step forward, she reveled in the congratulatory attention we all gave her. Now that she is an adult, we continue to celebrate milestones, such as taking the public transit system alone, or using her bank card to make a purchase on her own.

Before you became a parent, you may not have heard the terms *developmental milestones, gross motor,* or *fine motor.* As your nurturing relationship with your child grows with each passing day, you will gradually learn a whole new vocabulary of medical, developmental, and therapy words.

To understand what this book is all about, you need to understand the distinction between the two types of motor (movement) skills that your child will develop. ***Gross motor*** refers to the development of larger movements, such as those necessary for sitting and walking. ***Fine motor*** refers to the development of small muscle movements in the hands. When we think of fine motor skills, usually we think of activities such as tying our shoes, printing, or stringing beads. These are all fine motor skills, but they are the end result of a lot of preparation that has been going on in the child's muscles and nervous system.

Development occurs along a continuum, and our hands are not separate from the rest of our body. Therefore, fine motor skills develop in the context of the development of the whole child, including mobility, cognitive, social, language, and emotional development.

The "House" Model of Fine Motor Skills

The development of fine motor skills is like the construction of a house. The first thing that is laid down is the foundation. This supports all the levels above it. The first floor provides additional support for the second floor, and so on. The foundation for the fine motor skills house consists of Stability, Bilateral Coordination, and Sensation/Sensory processing. The next level up is Dexterity. These foundations support the Daily Living Skills, such as dressing and other self-care activities, and school-related skills, such as printing. Achievement of daily living skills supports independent living and work skills in teens and adults.

This is the model of the fine motor skill "house" I will refer to:

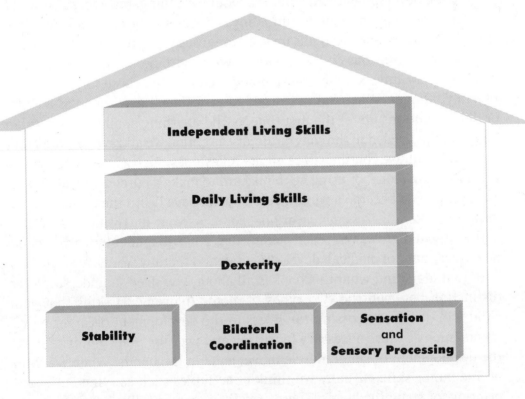

When a building is being constructed, workers never begin with the top floor. They lay the foundation, and then they can build the first floor, second floor, and so on. So it is with fine motor skills. During the early years, the "building blocks" are developing—the foundation upon which children can build the dexterity needed for daily living skills.

What Are the Building Blocks of Fine Motor Skills?

Stability	Bilateral Coordination	Sensation and Sensory Processing

What Is Stability?

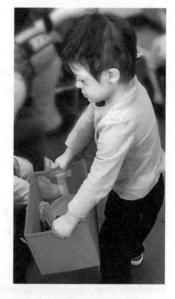

Stability is being able to push open a heavy door. Stability is being able to put on your shoes without falling over. It is carrying a tray full of drinks. It is holding a camera still while clicking a picture. In short, stability is a combination of strength and balance that enables us to keep one part of our body still while another part moves.

What Is Bilateral Coordination?

Bilateral coordination is holding the bowl with one hand while stirring with the other. It is holding the paper with one hand while cutting with scissors with the other. It is doing up your zipper and shoelaces. Bilateral coordination refers to the efficient use of both hands during an activity. Most daily activities require the coordinated use of both hands— one as the "doer" and the other as the "helper." Bilateral coordination leads eventually to the development of a dominant hand (becoming right or left handed).

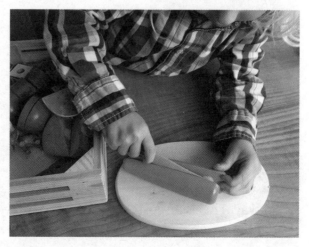

What Is Sensation?

Sensation is reaching into your pocket and leaving the Kleenex in while you take out the coins. It is putting a ponytail in your hair. It is knowing where to put your hands to catch a ball. Sensation is knowing where your fingers, hands, and arms are, and how they are moving, without constant conscious attention to them.

We all know the five senses: vision, hearing, smell, taste, and touch. We also have two other senses:

- **Proprioception**—the sense of joint position and movement, perceived by nerves in the joints, tendons, and muscles;
- **Vestibular system**—the sense that tells us the direction and speed of movement and position of our head in relation to gravity.

Chapter 7 focuses on the senses we use to develop coordinated movement, specifically fine motor movement. These are the senses of touch, proprioception, and vision.

What Is Sensory Processing?

Sensory processing is being able to play in a sandbox with other children, without distress about the feel of the sand or others being close and occasionally touching you. Sensory processing is coordinating balance, vision, and arm movements in order to hit a tennis ball with a racquet. Sensory processing is the ability to run around at recess, then line up, go inside, and sit at a desk.

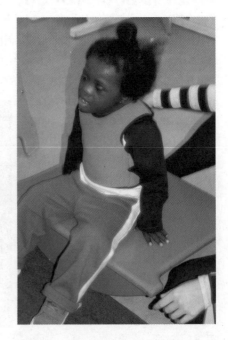

Sensory processing refers to the neural processes of registering, modulating, interpreting, and integrating all the information coming in from all the senses together, so that we can respond in an adaptive, functional way. This is discussed in Chapter 11.

The Second Level in the Hand Skills House: Dexterity

Your child begins to develop the building blocks for fine motor skill development at birth, and continues to do so for several years. As soon as he is able to grasp a toy placed in his hand (usually between three and six months), he begins the process of developing dexterity, which also progresses and develops for many years. All the while, the building blocks continue to lay the foundation and support the development of fine hand movements. In other words, the "building blocks" (stability, bilateral coordination, and sensation/ sensory processing) continue to be refined while the next level in the house, dexterity, begins to take shape.

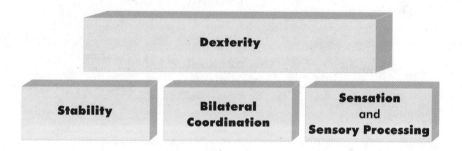

What Is Dexterity?

Dexterity is picking up a crayon and positioning it in your hand to color. It is opening a jar. Dexterity is opening and closing a safety pin. It is picking up a raisin. It is threading a needle. Dexterity enables us to make small, precise, accurate, and efficient movements with our hands without tremendous effort. When your child has established some of the foundations and is developing dexterity, he is able to use these abilities in his daily living skills.

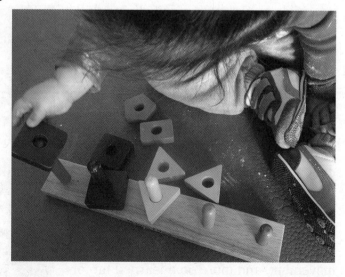

The Third Level in the Hand Skills House: Daily Living Skills

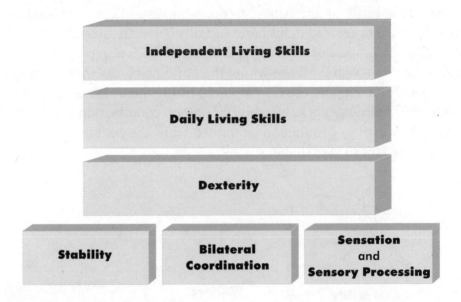

What Are Daily Living Skills?

Getting dressed in the morning is a daily living skill. Feeding ourselves is a daily living skill. Participating in classroom learning is a daily living skill. For children, playing is a daily living skill. Our children participate in different types of functional skills every day:

School tasks related to fine motor development include preprinting, printing, drawing and coloring, cutting, writing, and computer and technology skills. These are sometimes referred to as visual motor skills, because the child coordinates vision with his hand movements to learn these skills. As these skills mature, the movements can become more automatic, relying less on vision to guide the movement, and more on a learned motor movement. For example, someone who has learned to type well doesn't have to look at each finger before pressing the key.

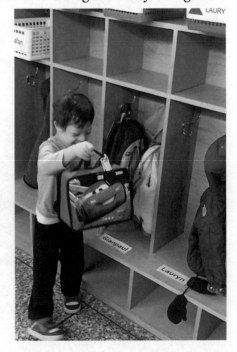

Self-help skills are all the activities we do on a routine, daily basis to take care of our bodies, and include dressing, eating, and grooming.

Household tasks and leisure activities are hobbies, play activities, sports pastimes, and routine household activities and chores that are part of the everyday life of adults and children.

What Are Independent Living Skills?

Preparing a meal is an independent living skill. Using an ATM machine is an independent living skill. Making a phone call, or sending a text or email is an independent living skill. Independent living skills are all the things we do in our lives as adults. Independent Living skills as they relate to fine motor skills will be briefly discussed in Chapter 10.

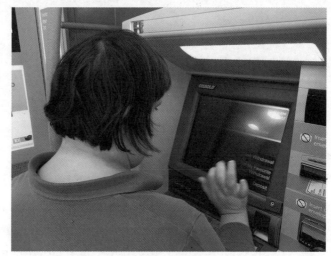

Putting on the Finishing Touches

The basic structure of the "fine motor skills house" goes up quickly, but all the finishing touches take years to develop and refine. The building blocks provide the foundation, and dexterity provides the specific movements upon which daily living skills can develop. Repeated practice of some of the daily living skills can "feed back" to improve dexterity and reinforce the foundation skills. It is like an electrical current in the wiring of a house; it travels in both directions.

Let us look at an example of how a daily living skill depends on and has an impact all the way through the "house model," shown on the next page.

In the construction of any house, the finishing touches seem to take the longest to complete. There are endless details: painting and wallpapering, tiles, light fixtures, kitchen cabinets and fixtures, doors, etc. So it is with the hand skills house. The refinement of all the skills on the "upper floors," all the details of development to make everything work "right," takes years to complete. For example, although your child will probably begin to finger feed himself around his first birthday, he will not have refined his eating skills (including cutting and spreading with a knife) until mid- to late childhood.

The development of fine motor skills begins in early infancy and continues until adulthood. Your awareness of how these skills develop will help you choose activities to do at home that will help your child continue to improve his fine motor abilities.

2

Building on What Is There:
Learning Step by Step

When Sarah was about eight years old, I decided to try to teach her our phone number. (I felt it was important for safety and social reasons for her to know her own phone number.) For several months I tried now and then (not very consistently, I might add), with little success. She just couldn't seem to get it. While she remembered some of the numbers, she would mix them up, forget the rest, skip some, and repeat others. Unfortunately, knowing some of the numbers some of the time doesn't help in an emergency.

When we both had more time in the summer, I decided to focus on it a bit more. I made up index cards with the individual numbers of our phone number written on them. We laid them down on the floor in order, numbers showing, and made a hopscotch game out of them. As Sarah jumped from square to square, she called out the numbers. Gradually we were able to turn some, then all, of the cards over. Sarah could now jump and call out the numbers by memory. After a couple of weeks of consistent practice, she could remember her phone number without the cues she first had (visual cues: seeing the numbers on the cards; and motor cues: jumping).

In looking back at my initial attempts to teach Sarah, I can come up with several reasons why I wasn't successful:

1. **She wasn't ready.** Children with Down syndrome need help to learn new skills, but they also need to be "ready." Being ready means that their nervous system development, their cognitive abilities, and their motor control have developed sufficiently to allow them to learn that particular skill. Sometimes we won't know

that a child isn't ready until we try something. If the child cannot seem to grasp the ultimate goal of the activity, then she isn't ready. For example, you may give her a few small blocks and demonstrate stacking them. After many demonstrations over several days, she continues to toss the blocks over the edge of the table and watch them fall. She is at the stage of understanding object permanence—knowing that the blocks do not disappear, that they fall and land on the floor. She is not quite ready to stack them!

2. **She wasn't interested or motivated.** Motivation is a strong driving force. Once a new teaching strategy was introduced, Sarah was more motivated to learn her phone number. Another motivation could have been a desire to share her phone number with new friends. The skill has to have some meaning and relevance to engage the child in the repetition needed for learning.

3. **She wasn't able to pay attention long enough to learn.** Children with Down syndrome may be easily distracted and may have difficulty attending in order to learn. This ties in with being "ready." If the activity is too far beyond her cognitive level, she won't be able to attend well. Auditory attention and memory weakness result in the child having difficulty processing and remembering verbal information.

4. **She learned better with a multisensory approach.** Remembering what they hear is very difficult for most children with Down syndrome (this is called auditory memory). Research and the experience of professionals who teach children with Down syndrome have found that they are usually "visual learners"; that is, they learn better when information and skills are taught visually, or with a combination of visual and auditory presentations. Sarah needed to see and hear the numbers over and over. She also needed to be active physically (jumping) to help her remember.

5. **The repetition wasn't consistent and frequent enough.** Children with Down syndrome need much more time and repetition to learn a new skill or ability. Short, frequent exposure to the activity may be more beneficial than longer, less frequent experiences.

If we are trying to help our child learn any new skill, we must start at the level she is at today. We must learn to expect small steps at a time. We must make sure that what we are trying to teach is meaningful to her; that is, she can see the point in doing it. If it is meaningful, it will be motivating. If we keep these things in mind, we learn to recognize every tiny step as a step forward, keeping us and our child motivated to continue trying.

Steps in Learning Skills

Much of your child's learning will take place through exploration, play, and interaction with her environment and with the primary people in it. Young children with Down syndrome need opportunities to learn through both structured and unstructured play experiences. Your child needs many opportunities to be self-directed in her unstructured play, which will expand her capabilities to initiate and follow through with planned actions. Most early intervention and infant development programs provide sequential skill guidelines for parents and caregivers to follow in order to facilitate the acquisition of the next stage of development and provide a structured approach to learning through play. Understandably, most parents try to help their child learn the developmental skills that are next on the list.

Here is an example of an infant development activity:

"The child watches the parent place a small toy in a box and opens the box to retrieve the toy." This activity relates to the child's understanding of the concept of object permanence. That is, she recognizes that even though the toy is temporarily out of sight, it is still there, and she can figure out how to get it. There are many other ways that the child can demonstrate this skill. For example, she can uncover a toy hidden by a blanket in her crib, or she can reach for the keys that you have put in your purse. The point is it is not always necessary to teach the precise skill as outlined, if you can see that the general concept and understanding is present in your child's spontaneous actions and play.

The understanding of how children with Down syndrome learn has evolved. In the past, it was generally believed that all of their learning followed the typical pattern, but was significantly slowed down. This concept has been broadened to a recognition of differences in the neurological underpinnings of learning. Learning of new skills takes place in a social context. According to Jennifer Wishart, a researcher in the United Kingdom, children with Down syndrome may develop a learning style that is characterized by "increasing use of avoidance strategies, a growing reluctance to take initiative in learning contexts, and an over-dependence on/misuse of social skills in cognitive contexts" (84).* In my experience, attempting to teach fine motor skills in an overly structured, adult-driven format may result in some of the above behaviors being exhibited. However, incorporating the same skill incorporated into a different context sometimes results in more engagement and less "learned helplessness" from the child.

When you are trying to help your child learn a new skill, there are a variety of considerations to keep in mind:

- the amount of support required,

---

* Numbers in parentheses refer to references at the back of the book.

- the type of support required,
- the level of interest and engagement by the child, and
- your responses to your child's learning attempts.

These considerations are part of the dynamic interplay of the learning partnership.

Amount of Support
full assistance
partial assistance
no assistance: independent

Type of Support
physical assistance
visual supports
verbal support / emotional support

LEARNING PARTNERSHIP

Child Engagement
uninterested
limited engagement
attentive, engaged
motivated, persists at task

Social Context
learning history of child
responses of learning partners
peer interactions
learning expectations:
too high or too low?

It can be helpful to think of these interconnected dynamics in a progression, being aware that every child may not follow step by step, and that the social context is also important.

These are the steps we go through with our children with Down syndrome when helping them learn how to do things for themselves:

1. **Uninterested:** Your child is dependent on you to do the whole activity because she is unable to participate yet.

2. **Watches adult/peer modeling:** Your child watches and shows interest in the activity but does not yet participate.

3. **Physical assistance:** Your child can start to participate but needs physical assistance to complete the activity. Sometimes hand-over-hand help gives the child a "feel" for how to do the activity. A lot of children dislike hand-over-hand help, however, and prefer to try on their own. This can be a

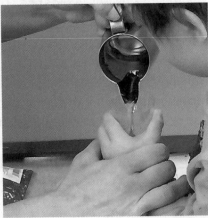

challenging stage for you, as your child struggles to attempt the activity but refuses your help.

4. **Physical and verbal assistance:** Your child can do part of the activity without hand-over-hand assistance but still needs us to talk her through it and to help physically with some of the activity.

5. **Verbal and/or visual assistance:** Your child can complete the activity without any physical help, but needs to be talked through it, with specific verbal instruction or needs to follow visual prompts, such as sequential pictures of each step of the task.

6. **Emotional support:** Your child can do the activity herself, without physical or instructional help but needs the emotional support of your presence. ("You're doing a great job, keep going, you're almost done," etc.)

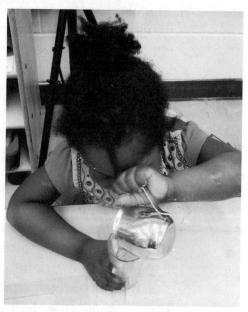

7. **Independent:** Your child can do the activity completely independently. She then practices the skill over and over until it is consolidated. Until she has had sufficient practice, the skill is not fully learned, and will not be consistent from day to day.

8. **Generalization of skill:** Only once the skill is fully consolidated into your child's automatic repertoire of skills will she be able to generalize it to other situations. For example, a young child may learn to drink from one particular cup at home, but seem unable to generalize this skill to a different cup at preschool. The skill is not yet automatic, and the child depends on some of the familiar aspects of drinking (perhaps the color or shape of the cup, or the highchair she sits in, or even how the cup is handed to her) to trigger the appropriate motor response. When she can drink out of any cup in any environment, she has generalized that skill. Sometimes children learn a skill at school, but don't do it at home, and vice versa. The skill has not yet been generalized to the other environment. Generalization of skills may not come automatically for some children with Down syndrome, and the skill may need to be taught in each environment.

Let's apply these steps in learning to a specific skill: tying shoelaces.

1. You tie your child's shoelaces. She is not really interested and her gaze wanders around the room.
2. You tie your child's shoelaces. Now she is interested, watching your movements.
3. Your child is at a developmental age when it is appropriate to begin to learn to tie shoelaces. She is already untying her laces. She can hold the laces with both hands, but can't move through the sequence of movements without your help.
4. Your child knows how to do some of the tying, such as doing the initial knot and making the "bunny ears" with your verbal cues, but she still needs some physical prompting to cross and tie the bunny ears and pull them tight.
5. Your child can manage the physical aspects of the activity with verbal prompts, such as "cross over, then under," or visual prompts to see the various steps.
6. Your child manages the activity, needing your emotional support to set it up and complete—for example, "You're doing great; you've done one foot, only one more to go!" She may continue to benefit from visual prompts.
7. Your child can tie her laces without your assistance. She then is expected to tie them consistently, with your understanding that some days she may go back to needing some assistance or support, as the skill will not be totally consistent until she has had sufficient practice. For children with Down syndrome, sufficient practice may be more practice than for the typically developing child.
8. Your child can consistently tie her shoelaces on different pairs of shoes, in a variety of situations, such as at home, before gym class, at a community program, etc. The skill has been consolidated, and it is automatic.

Here is another example of the steps involved in learning a specific activity: printing her name.

1. The teacher/parent prints your child's name on her paper.
2. Your child watches as her name is printed, perhaps repeating the names of the letters as they are printed.
3. Your child attempts to print her name, needing some physical guidance to do so. Remember, it is not necessary that the letters be formed perfectly at this stage! In fact, correct letter formation comes with a lot of practice (see Chapter 9).

4. Your child prints part of her name, but needs some physical guidance or physical demonstration, and also verbal cuing.

5. Your child prints most or all of her name, but needs to be talked through it: "What letter comes next?" "Remember how we make an L? Start at the top, make a line down; that's right, now go across. Good!"

6. Your child can print her name, but needs assurance and feedback along the way.

7. Your child prints her name on her own. Hooray! Now she practices printing it until it becomes automatic.

8. Once printing her name is automatic, your child will generalize her ability and will be able to print her name with any kind of writing tool, in any kind of situation (e.g., on the top of a worksheet, in a greeting card, etc.).

Bear in mind that it often takes years for a child with Down syndrome to move through the eight steps with some activities, as in the example of learning to print her name. She may begin to learn at age four, and may reach the stage of being able to print her name completely independently at age eight. It's easy to be out of sync with your child with these learning steps. When Sarah was learning to dress herself, I had to remind myself that it was okay that I had to be there to talk Sarah through getting dressed every morning; at least I didn't usually have to guide her through it physically any more. On the other hand, your child might sometimes be ready to move on to the next step, but you are so used to helping her, or helping her more than she needs, that you don't step back and let her try. It's a fine line!

When we describe abilities in children with Down syndrome, bear in mind that developmental assessments or checklists with an "able/unable" or "pass/fail" approach will not capture all those stages in between that our children may be in for so long. Assessments that are more descriptive, or that break the skills down into levels of independence, will probably be more useful for parents and teachers in program planning.

Accepting Inconsistency

It's all right to expect your child to do more at certain times than at others. I have learned that "inconsistent" describes Sarah's abilities. For example, when she was first learning to print, some days she could pull it all together and print her name legibly. But other days she reversed or missed letters and couldn't correct them, even if she recognized her errors. We all have good days and bad days. Our children's abilities on a particular day are related to so many internal and external factors, such as motivation, interest, fatigue, etc. Our child's ability to interpret and respond to sensory information from the environment (sensory processing) can vary from situation to situation and day to day. As parents, the best we can do is to try to be tuned in to our child's "state," so we can judge what to expect of her. This variability in performance within one child has been noted by professionals and researchers working with children with Down syndrome (84).

It takes longer for children with Down syndrome to learn things, and attention and short-term memory deficits complicate the learning process. Sometimes, even when they seem to have learned a skill, they can't always recall it from their memory. They can't seem to make the connections to enable the skill to come out. Then the next day they have no problem. Although this might be interpreted as "stubborn behavior," it can sometimes be a failure of the sensory-motor pathways to make the right neural connections all the time. Most of the time the connection happens, sometimes it doesn't, and as frustrated as we can be with it, imagine how frustrating and demoralizing it can be for the child. She has worked so hard to learn a skill, seems to have learned it, and then can't do it the next day. In this situation, using a visual or verbal prompts that was part of the initial learning process may help trigger the learned response.

Motivation

Your child's approach to learning will relate to her unique personality, health, previous experiences, relationships, abilities, and sensory preferences. Patricia Winders, in her book *Gross Motor Skills in Children with Down Syndrome* (83), noted that young children with Down syndrome who are learning motor skills tend to be either "motor driven" or "observers." That is, some children want to plunge right in and try a new skill as soon as they can, and other children prefer to watch and wait, and need more encouragement. In addition, research has begun to help us understand the *differences* in learning as experienced by children with Down syndrome as compared to other children. We are starting to understand that it is not always simply a delay in learning (81, 84). Parents, teachers, and educational assistants sometimes struggle with the typical package of parenting and teaching strategies, which may not always be as successful for the child with Down syndrome.

Motivation is critical for engagement of your child in the activity. Any child will show more interest in activities that are "fun" than in those that are presented or perceived as "exercises" or "therapy." A baby's and young child's primary means of learning about the world around her and of developing her abilities are through play and social interaction. "Fun" is, however, a very subjective thing. We have all heard about children who have more fun playing with the cardboard box than with the expensive toy that came in it. What is "fun" depends on a multitude of factors, including personality, age, and culture.

For example, let's consider the child who is learning how to stack objects on top of each other. When we attempt to teach the child this skill with blocks, the child more often than not just wants to knock down the blocks. However, she is happy to stack the rolls of toilet paper one on top of another in the bathroom cabinet. Or consider the child who has learned to pick up a toy with one hand and pass it to the other hand (*transferring*). She is now ready to pick up two objects simultaneously with each hand and bring them together in midline (the center of her body). Picking up two wooden cube blocks and banging them together may not be particularly motivating to this child. She may, however, be quite interested in holding a pot lid and banging it with a wooden spoon, or in banging toy cymbals together and making a racket!

When choosing fine motor activities that will be motivating for your child, consider the following points (which are based on my experience and that of researchers and other professionals):

1. Have Realistic Expectations: Know what stage your child is at, and what comes next. This book will help you understand the sequence of fine motor development. You will know if the activity is either too challenging physically or intellectually, or isn't enough of a challenge for your child, by her response. If she is totally unable to participate in the activity, even with your help, the activity is probably too difficult right now. Persisting at skills that are beyond your child's current developmental readiness will result in frustration in both you and your child.

Bear in mind that your child may not give you signs that she is ready for more challenging activities, or the next stage of an activity. Some children with Down syndrome are quite happy to participate in play and other activities that are at an earlier developmental level than what they are capable of. She may need structure and prompting to move on to the next stage.

2. Build on Success: Use activities that you know your child has had success with. Build on that success by adding a bit more difficulty to an already accomplished activity. For example, if your child can pour milk from a very small pitcher into her cereal bowl and enjoys doing so, progress to pouring from gradually larger pitchers into gradually smaller cups. Success and accomplishment are inherently motivating. The emotional connection to successfully interacting with the environment through a self-initiated activity enhances learning (30, 86).

3. Break Down the Activity into Small Steps: Remember the stages of learning already discussed in this chapter. Learn to be rewarded by every small step your child is able to make. For example, we don't hand a child a crayon and expect her to color a picture inside the lines the first time! First we expect scribbling all over the page, then scribbling oriented to the space where the picture is, then some awareness of coloring the picture itself, with a gradual refinement and control of the crayon stroke until it can be recognized as "coloring in the lines."

4. Make It "Fun": I have certainly found that taking a personal approach with Sarah and the other children I have worked with greatly influences their interest in trying and persisting at an activity. Be very aware of your voice and body language, as they can be powerful tools to help motivate your child. Using a silly voice or building a game out of an activity takes more ingenuity and creativity on your part, but it can pay off. Don't forget to take your turn during any kind of game! Turn-taking is an important social interaction skill, and reinforces your own interest in the activity.

5. Make It Relevant: We all know that it is hard to keep at something that is difficult when it doesn't seem important or relevant to our lives. It is the same for our children. Many things that we take for granted will have to be taught to our children with Down syndrome, and will be difficult at first. For example, your child may not see the point of doing up buttons on a button board in the classroom every day for ten minutes. However, she may see the point in buttoning her sweater before recess so she can go outside to play. If your child can practice fine motor skills at times of the day and during routines that make sense and have meaning for her, she will likely be more motivated to try. Also, it doesn't always follow that a child who can do up buttons on a button board will be able to do up her own buttons. She may not be able to generalize her ability with a skill in one setting or with one piece of equipment to other settings or objects. Children with Down syndrome need to learn the skills needed for daily activities by practicing those exact activities.

6. Be Aware of the Environment: Learning new skills requires attention and focus. Be aware of distractions that may interfere with your child's attempts at the activity. Other aspects to be aware of in terms of optimal learning are time of day, energy level, hunger and hydration, physical space, seating, interruptions, background noise, and lighting. Be aware of the sensory aspects of the activity and how they may be affecting your child's interest. Your child's processing of the sensory aspects of the environment may affect her learning ability on any given day.

7. Try it! If it doesn't work, you can always try something else!

What motivates your child? What is she interested in? What is a meaningful reward for her for trying to learn a new skill? As parents, we often know the answers to these questions intuitively, but we may not always listen to these intuitions as we try to teach our child what we think, or others think, she "should" be doing. Many children are unenthusiastic about trying activities that they perceive as difficult, in which they expect to fail. It is important to reinforce all the efforts your child makes and to show her that it's all right to make mistakes, so that she doesn't develop a perception of failure. We all need time and practice to learn new things. Let your child know that.

Adapting the Environment

Making changes and adaptations to the environment can also be important in helping to build your child's success with fine motor skills. This is an important component of occupational therapy practice: ensuring the best possible fit between the person and environment. For example, adapting an infant's seat to promote better positioning for hand play would be considered adapting the environment. Using clothing with a minimum of fastenings to make independent dressing easier for a child is another example.

The environment includes the physical and sensory attributes and the social aspects of the places the child spends time in. All contribute to a child's sense of safety, well-being, and readiness to learn. Children with intellectual disabilities are more vulnerable to the state of the environment. Aspects of the environment can have both a positive and negative impact on them. For an infant, the environment includes her home and possibly day care center or babysitter's home. For an older child, the environment is her home, school, day care, camp, community recreation center, etc. For an adult, the environment may include home, work, social programs, place of worship, etc.

"Adapting the environment" means *changing, eliminating, or adding something* so the child can be more independent or successful. For example, a nine-year-old boy requested drinks from his mother several times a day. His mother made two changes that made it possible for him to get his own drinks. She began putting the juice in smaller jugs in the fridge, so they would not be too heavy for him to pour. She also moved the cups to a shelf in a lower cupboard, so he could reach them himself.

In another example, a four-year-old child with Down syndrome continues to hold crayons and markers clenched in her palm when coloring. Instead of markers, she could be given short stubs of crayons or chalk, which promote

the use of a three-finger (tripod) grasp. In addition, drawing at an upright easel or paper board would encourage her to use more mature wrist and hand positioning.

"Adapting the environment" can also include making changes to the sensory aspect of the environment. A child who quickly becomes overstimulated and distracted by a preschool room full of toys and activities may be more successful in a room where she can choose between only a few activities at a time.

For children with Down syndrome, body position can be crucial to success with fine motor skills. Sometimes adding support for the child's body position is all that is needed to adapt the environment so the child can do the activity. For instance, when she was about seven years old, Sarah had a Mickey Mouse watch that talked and told the time when both sides of the watch were pressed simultaneously. The watch required a fair amount of pressure to activate, and she was unable to do it without taking note of her body position. She learned that she had to place her elbow and forearm down on a firm surface to give her enough stability and strength to make Mickey talk. Due to low muscle tone and joint hypermobility, children with Down syndrome need close attention to body position when they are doing fine motor activities.

Consultation with an Occupational Therapist

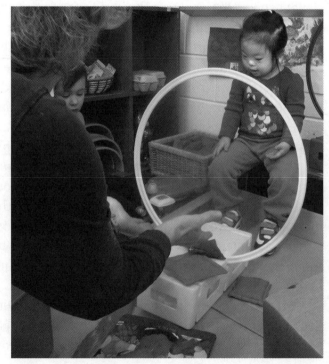

This book was designed to give parents, teachers, and others general guidance in 1) encouraging the development of fine motor skills in children with Down syndrome and 2) understanding the role of sensory processing on the development of their child. In developing these skills, many infants and children with Down syndrome can benefit from the services of an occupational therapist at some point in their life.

What Is an Occupational Therapist?

Occupational therapists are professionals who promote independence in daily living skills in clients of all ages when a physical, developmental, or psychosocial challenge interferes with the person's abilities. "Occupational" refers to the occupations people perform throughout their daily life, which for children include self-care, leisure, play, and school activities. Promotion of independence occurs within the context of the person's environment and relationships.

An occupational therapist (OT) has at least a four-year college or university degree with courses in sciences, typical development, medical and mental health conditions, and the theory and practice of occupational therapy. An occupational therapist can become involved with you and your child either through direct intervention or through consultation, and will focus on your child's ability to interact with her environment in ways that lead to mastery and independence. An occupational therapist can be a resource for both parents and teachers, can provide information about neurological and sensory-motor development, and can assess the physical and sensory environment in relation to the child's abilities.

Children with Down syndrome may receive occupational therapy services through an infant development or early intervention program, in a clinic or hospital setting, and in preschools and schools. Some occupational therapists are in private practice. The national associations of occupational therapy listed in the Resources section of this book can provide guidance in finding an occupational therapist for your child.

How Can Occupational Therapy Help Your Child?

For children with Down syndrome, OT involvement may be directed at helping with the following:

- self-care skills (eating, dressing, grooming, etc.);
- fine and gross motor skills;
- skills related to school performance (e.g., printing, cutting, etc.);
- play, leisure, and work skills;
- sensory processing needs

During infancy, an occupational therapist may become involved with you and your child to assist with the following:

- Positioning and feeding techniques related to oral motor and feeding difficulties. Sometimes sensory issues around feeding need to be addressed by an OT.
- Gross motor and fine motor milestones, particularly fine motor skills. Physical therapists work to encourage proper movement patterns for mobility and the development of gross motor skills.

Occupational therapists promote arm and hand movement patterns and milestones that lay the foundation for refined fine motor skills.

During the toddler and preschool years, an occupational therapist may be involved for these reasons:

- To facilitate the development of fine motor skills through play and specific activities to develop control of isolated hand movements (dexterity), such as turning knobs and pushing buttons on toys, and building with construction and stacking toys;
- To observe the child in her environment(s) (e.g., home, day care, or preschool), paying attention to the child-environment "fit" and the sensory needs of the child;
- To help parents and caregivers promote the beginning steps of self-help skills such as eating, drinking, and dressing. An OT can help parents set appropriate expectations, as well as help with positioning and suggestions for specialized equipment and adaptations.

During the school years, an occupational therapist may be involved in these areas:

- Providing direct intervention to your child to help her learn visual-motor skills such as preprinting and printing and consulting with the teacher about printing learning methods, adaptations, positioning, appropriate fine motor expectations, etc. Some occupational therapists have expertise in assistive technology, such as computer adaptations, that can be of benefit to the child in the classroom.
- Helping to set realistic expectations for the continued learning of self-help skills.
- Helping your child develop specific fine motor skills that will lead to more success in school and self-help activities.
- Addressing any sensory processing needs that may be interfering with your child's interactions and learning.

As our children grow up and eventually leave school, they will enter new work and social environments. At this stage, an occupational therapist may be involved with the following:

- Evaluating the components of a job your child is being considered for and her ability to perform them.
- Helping her master independent living skills.

- Evaluating physical or sensory challenges to daily living skills, and suggesting strategies and adaptations to minimize the effects of those challenges.

Parents Know Their Child Best

Occupational therapists and other professionals have expertise and can provide guidance and therapeutic intervention, and they can help you understand the particular challenges your child faces. They can also point you in the direction of important resources in your community. However, *you* are the expert on your child. You know your child best, her temperament, what helps calm her, what excites and motivates her, etc. The relationship between you and the professionals in your life is ideally as members of a mutually respectful team. Your thoughts and opinions are of utmost importance and so are your questions. I have learned so much as an occupational therapist by listening to my daughters, the children I work with, and their parents.

Some adaptations, such as the example of the juice jug and cups given above, can be thought up by parents if they ask themselves, "Is there any way I can make this activity easier or more efficient for my child and myself?" Many parents and teachers make these changes automatically, without thinking of it as "adapting the environment." Observing and being aware of your child is the first step to recognizing how a difficult or dependent situation can possibly be changed so your child has more independence.

Depending on the social and cultural environment, adults may think there is only one "right" way of doing things. By keeping an open mind, we can see that there are choices about how to do things, and we can choose the way that is best for our child right now.

3

Fine Motor Development in Children with Down Syndrome

This chapter describes common aspects of Down syndrome that can affect a child's development of fine motor abilities. Understanding how and why Down syndrome affects your child's fine motor skills can help you determine both when to introduce an activity and when not to push. It can also help you to recognize whether your child needs adaptations to accomplish a skill. In addition, it can help you understand the difficulties your child is having and determine whether they are typical for a child with Down syndrome.

Later chapters will discuss how we can try to help our children overcome these difficulties as much as possible in order to learn fine motor skills that are important in their daily lives. In this chapter, the developing fine motor skills are outlined for each age range, using the house model that was introduced in Chapter 1.

How Does Down Syndrome Affect Fine Motor Skill Development?

Each child with Down syndrome develops fine motor skills at his own pace and has his own individual strengths and needs. Development of motor skills progresses from large joints (those closer to the body) to small joints (those further away). Control of movement develops first in the shoulder, then elbow, then wrist, then fingers and thumb. This is called proximal to distal development. In addition, there are a variety of characteristics associated with Down syndrome that can affect fine motor skill development. These include physical characteristics (such as hypotonia), medical problems, and cognitive delays.

Physical Characteristics
Hypotonia

Hypotonia or *low muscle tone* is lower than normal tension in the muscles. Our muscles always have some degree of contraction, even if we are not moving, as they hold our bones in place. Children with Down syndrome have varying degrees of low muscle tone. This makes them appear floppy and delays the development of head and body control.

Any child with hypotonia has difficulty with the first developmental motor challenge of learning to move into upright positions. Holding up his head, propping up on his arms, lifting his hands and feet into the air, sitting, etc.—all of these skills are slower to develop because the infant can't activate enough tone in his muscles to move into a more upright position, and, if he is placed upright, to hold that position.

In children with Down syndrome, hypotonia affects all the muscles of the body. Thus, our children have low muscle tone in their tongue and face, fingers and hands, as well as in their torso, arms, and legs. Just as low muscle tone affects their gross motor development, so too does it affect their fine motor development.

A child who is struggling to keep his balance in sitting because of low muscle tone in his body will be less able to reach out and pick up toys. Low muscle tone in the shoulder and upper back area also impair the baby's ability to reach and grasp (78). Likewise, low muscle tone in the lower arm and hand make it difficult for the child to position his finger joints to hold an object such as a pencil without his joints "collapsing." It may be particularly difficult for the child to push with his fingers, such as when pushing a button on a pop-up toy or pushing a thumbtack into a bulletin board. The muscles in the hand may not have enough tone to stabilize the joints.

Generally, the literature suggests that hypotonia in children with Down syndrome decreases with age. The problem is that by then, they may have developed ways of moving that may be detrimental in the stages of motor development that follow. For example, a child with Down syndrome who dislikes being on his stomach may eventually learn to move himself around the room on his back or his bottom by pushing and pulling with his feet. If he never has the experience of leaning, pushing, and pulling himself on the floor with his arms, his shoulder muscles and arms may not have the amount of stability for things like pulling himself up to standing, and for fine control of movements such as eating soup or printing.

Ligament and Joint Laxity

The ligaments supporting the joints are also looser, allowing more movement at the joints; this is called *"hyperextension,"* or *"ligamentous laxity."* This increased range of movement in the joints is often very evident in our children's hands, especially when they are young. The thumb in particular may have so much extra movement that it is very difficult for the child to hold and manipulate smaller objects (87). A person without Down syndrome who has some joints that are "double jointed" can usually produce this excessive movement at will and has control over when it happens. The child with Down syndrome, however, cannot control the excessive joint movement.

Due to laxity around joint capsules, children with Down syndrome could have greater risk of joint subluxation or dislocation. Care must be taken not to pull excessively on your child's limbs. For example, if a young child who can't yet stand up from the floor independently is pulled up by his hands, it may put too much force on the joint structures of the shoulders and elbows. If there are any indications that your child may have a subluxed or dislocated joint, such as persistent pain around the joint, awkward positioning of a limb, or a tendency to avoid using a limb, he should be seen by a doctor.

Atlanto-Axial Instability

All parents of children with Down syndrome should be aware of a condition called atlanto-axial instability. In this condition, the first and second vertebrae of the spine, in the neck, are unstable due to lax ligaments. It is estimated that 10 to 30 percent of children with Down syndrome have this instability evident on x-ray; however, a much smaller percentage (1 to 2 percent) develop symptoms. When a child has this instability, extreme movement or force to the head or neck may result in injury to the spinal cord.

It is generally recommended that children with Down syndrome have a neck x-ray by the age of three to five to determine their risk for atlanto-axial instability. Children, teens, and adults of all ages should be checked before they sign up for sports activities where there is a risk of falling and injuring the neck (such as horseback riding or gymnastics). Some symptoms of atlanto-axial instability include neck pain, difficulty walking, incontinence, and decreased coordination. Atlanto-occipital instability is much rarer, but potentially more serious.

Shorter Limbs

You may have noticed that your child's arms and legs appear shorter than other children's relative to his torso. This is quite common in children with Down syndrome. This shorter length will be most noticeable when you are trying to help him learn to sit and to go into the hands-and-knees position.

(This is discussed in more detail on page 52.) When your child is a little older, you may also notice the shorter arm and leg length when you are trying to find a tricycle or bicycle to fit, and when buying clothing. Because your child has a little further to reach, tasks such as putting on and fastening shoes may be more challenging for his balance.

Hand Characteristics

Our children's hands may also have some unique physical characteristics:

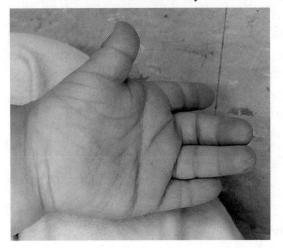

1. **Single Simean Crease:** Instead of having three creases in their palms, some children with Down syndrome have two. This is one of the signs used in making the diagnosis of Down syndrome at birth. There is no indication in the literature that this has any effect on hand function.

2. **Smaller Hands:** In general, the hand of a child with Down syndrome is smaller than average, and the fingers are shorter. This may make it more difficult to grasp and hold larger objects, such as when opening a large jar or when catching a ball with one hand. Activities requiring large finger span, such as using a computer keyboard or playing guitar or piano, may also be more difficult.

3. **Wrist Bones:** There are seven small wrist bones in the hand. At birth, some children with Down syndrome do not have all of these bones, but they usually develop them by adolescence (24). The absence of one or more wrist bones may make it more difficult for babies and young children to stabilize their hands at the wrist as they are developing grasping patterns. For example, when a child learns to let go of blocks to build a tower, he stabilizes at the wrist to allow his fingers to open and release the block.

4. **Curved Fifth Finger:** The finger (usually the fifth finger in Down syndrome) may be curved inward (called "clinodactyly"), or it may always be slightly bent at the middle (second) joint (called "camptodactyly"). If your child has either of these conditions present in one or both hands, he can't straighten his finger, nor will you be able to straighten it by pulling on it. If you are very concerned about it, your child should be seen by an or-

thopedic specialist. In the general population, these two conditions of the fingers are sometimes managed by stretching and occasionally splinting (69). In my experience, children with Down syndrome who have this slightly unusual positioning of their fifth finger(s) do not receive stretching or splinting intervention. From a parent's perspective, it seems relatively minor, compared to some of the other challenges their child may face.

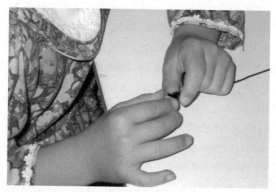

An example of clinodactyly in the little finger of the right hand.

Most people place the fifth finger side of their hand down on the table for stability when writing. Try writing with your fifth finger bent up and away from the rest of your hand, and feel the difference. I have seen this pattern of writing without the support of the fifth finger on the paper both in children who have clinodactyly or camptodactyly, and in those who don't. The effect of clinodactyly or camptodactyly on hand function in children with Down syndrome has not been studied, to my knowledge.

Medical Conditions

Most children with Down syndrome who also have a congenital heart condition experience even more difficulty achieving early developmental milestones. *Cardiac problems* impair stamina and endurance for motor activity. Many children with Down syndrome also have increased susceptibility to, and frequency of, infections due to a weaker immune system and structural differences (such as smaller nasal passages and ear canals). *Respiratory and ear infections*, in particular, are frequent. We know that when our children are ill, they have much less energy for anything, which affects their development.

Some children with Down syndrome have *visual problems* that may affect eye-hand coordination. In fact, some researchers estimate that 50 percent of people with Down syndrome have some type of visual error (77). Difficulties with visual acuity and coordination of the movements of the eyes can make it more difficult for the eyes and hands to work together in fine motor tasks. Many children with Down syndrome are "visual learners," meaning that vision is the dominant sense when they are learning and remembering information and skills. Vision assists our children in learning movement patterns. Since our children rely on vision, yet are at risk for eye and visual problems, their vision should be assessed regularly. It can be difficult to keep glasses on a young child who would benefit from correction of a visual error but doesn't understand the importance of keeping his glasses on. Using straps to keep the glasses securely in place can be helpful.

Cognitive Level

Fine motor and cognitive skills go hand in hand during the early stages of development. Early cognitive learning develops as children manipulate objects in their environment. For example, a baby learns by dropping objects that they always fall *down,* or that a toy hidden under a cloth is still there when he lifts up the cloth (*object permanence).* Delays in fine motor abilities can also delay a child's understanding of the world around him if he is unable to manipulate objects in a way that will help him learn.

Young children with Down syndrome need extra guidance, modeling, verbal cuing, and encouragement to learn fine motor skills (88). As a result, fine motor tasks that help the child learn cognitive concepts may have to be taught in a structured, systematic way. Like all children, our children with Down syndrome also benefit from opportunities to explore play materials in unstructured, self-directed ways.

As they progress through school, children with Down syndrome continue to use fine motor skills to express their developing understanding of materials and concepts through drawing and printing. Fine motor and visual motor difficulties may impede this expression of knowledge and understanding. For example, your school-aged child may understand that plants need sunlight, water, and soil to grow. But when asked to draw a picture of what plants need, he may not have the visual motor ability to put this down on paper.

Likewise, the development of cognitive ability can affect a child's acquisition of fine motor skills. A child's cognitive level can direct the way he uses his hands. For instance, although a child with Down syndrome may have the physical ability to put Megablocks together to build a structure, he may not initiate this activity on his own. He may not be at the developmental level of combining and taking apart building toys. He may choose instead to put the blocks in his mouth, bang two blocks together, or poke his finger in the holes. Although he may have the physical potential to develop his fine motor skills further, he may not be responsive to more advanced types of activities. In these situations, the challenge is to find activities that do interest the child and are cognitively appropriate in order to help develop his fine motor skills.

Fine Motor Skills to Look for as Your Child Grows

This section provides an overview of fine motor skills to watch for and encourage at the various stages of development. The material is presented in the house model to show the relationship between the building block foundation skills and the emerging higher level skills. The skills mentioned are based on the average development of children with Down syndrome, and reflect the kinds of activities we can expect many children to participate in by the *end* of each stage. Bear in mind that there is great variability in the age at which children with Down syndrome achieve developmental milestones.

This section will give you an introduction to the developmental sequence of fine motor skills. Subsequent chapters will give more detailed activity suggestions for each building block, dexterity, and the daily living skills.

Birth to 2 Years

Rapid changes take place during these first two years of life. Your child develops enough control of his body so that by the end of the first year, he may be able to sit up alone briefly, and by his second birthday, he may be able to pull up to stand and possibly take a few steps. He also starts to actively explore his world by picking up things, looking at them, and putting them in his mouth.

By the end of this stage, he will have developed better sensation in his hands to feel and learn about things, and thus will not need to put objects in his mouth as often. The three building blocks—stability, bilateral coordination, and sensation—are the main areas of development of fine motor skills at this stage, but your child will also be starting to develop the skills and movements needed for dexterity, such as picking up small things.

During this stage, many parents choose to introduce signs and gestures to encourage communication. In North America, signed English is usually the system chosen. Exact imitation of the sign by your child is not necessary, as some of the standard sign language hand positions may be too difficult for a young child. Rather, adapt the sign so that your child can easily do it. For example, at age two Sarah was unable to verbally indicate her toileting needs. The traditional sign (thumb between third and fourth finger in a fisted hand) was too hard for her, so we used a closed fist, moving back and forth.

As parents and caregivers, we usually respond when our child points or picks up a toy by naming it and describing it and what it does, etc. It is important to keep in mind that our child with Down syndrome may not be able to initiate these kinds of fine motor movements without our help at this stage. As a result, he may not hear as much of the labeling and simple descriptive language from us. Researchers have found that children with Down syndrome who *were* able to engage in more active fine motor play had better language comprehension a year later. They theorized that those babies who could more actively explore and manipulate objects would elicit more specific references to these objects by their parents (70).

You can help your baby by assisting him to pick up, hold, and explore toys, and to point to things around him, and by naming and describing these things for him. Listed in the house model below are the kinds of skills to work toward during this first stage. Subsequent chapters give detailed descriptions and suggestions for each area of development.

Birth to 2 Years House Model

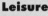

Leisure
Looks at picture books; Active play (riding toys);
Plays with toys

Self-Help
Starts to feed self with
fingers, spoon, cup;
Removes some clothing

Visual Motor
Scribbles with crayon

Dexterity
Reaches out to grasp; lets go with more and more control;
Puts things in/out of containers;
Points, pokes, isolates index finger;
Picks up small objects & explores them;
Waves bye-bye;
Uses hand gestures/signs for communication

Stability
Props on arms,
rocks on hands & knees;
Uses arms to move:
crawling, pulling
to stand;
Reaches in sitting;
Shakes toys

**Bilateral
Coordination**
Passes from one
hand to the other;
Uses both hands to play;
Takes apart toys such
as rings off peg;
Claps

Sensation
Looks at hands;
Wants to touch and
feel everything;
Brings toys to mouth;
Plays peek-a-boo

Preschooler: 2 to 4 Years

At this stage, your child will have developed much more control of his body. Although he is continuing to strengthen his "building blocks," he has developed them enough to begin to experiment with and practice many more movements with his hands. Dexterity begins to gradually take over from the building blocks as the primary focus of your child's hand skill development.

Using sign language to augment verbal communication helps your child learn to use his hands for meaningful activity and improves his dexterity. It

2 to 4 Years House Model

Leisure
Playgrounds;
Imaginary/dress-up play;
Rides toys/trike;
Looks at books

Self-Help
Uses a spoon;
Starts using a fork;
Puts cup down without spilling;
Pulls zipper up and down;
Takes off/puts on loose clothing

Visual Motor
Draws lines/circles/simple forms;
Holds scissors, snips;
Paints with brush;
Emerging tripod grasp of marker

Dexterity
Can let go of small objects more accurately;
Develops grasp: from holding in the palm to using fingers;
Can pick up small things;
Uses thumb and fingers to manipulate;
May use signs to augment communication;
Points with index finger;
Together-apart toys;
Uses simple apps/computer games

Stability
Uses arms for climbing (onto furniture, at playgrounds);
Plays with push/pull toys (wagons, carts);
Shovels sand/pours water;
Opens cupboards/closets

Bilateral Coordination
Hand preference begins to emerge;
Uses hands together to manipulate toys;
Holds toy steady when necessary while other hand manipulates

Sensation
Plays with sensory materials (play dough, sand);
Knows several body parts;
Puts things in mouth less often—explores with hands and eyes

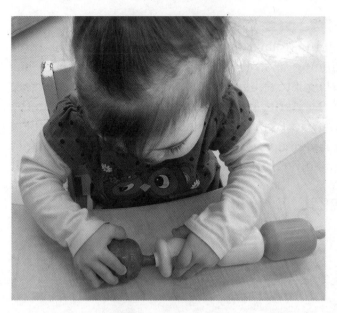

is also very important to help your child pick up objects and explore them by turning them around and over in his hands, looking at them, making them work by pushing buttons, etc. Sensory play—such as playing in sand or water or with finger paint, Play Doh, glue, and other sensory materials—is important at this stage. Other important play experiences at this stage include taking apart and putting together insert puzzles (the kind with the little knobs on each piece), manipulative toys such as Duplo, Tinkertoys, train sets, etc., toys with knobs and buttons (like pop-up toys), and toys for stacking, such as rings, pegs, and blocks. Your child will begin to participate actively in the routines of daily care, such as dressing, although he usually still needs considerable help.

Early School Aged: 5 to 8 Years

At this stage, when your child starts school, he will be using the dexterity skills he has already developed to learn more daily living skills, such as dressing and printing. He continues to develop coordination of the smaller muscles and joints in his hands, fingers, thumbs, and wrists. Your child will begin to handle routine tasks (such as dressing and toileting) more independently. As in previous stages, he will continue to strengthen the foundation skills; this increased strength will help him in new endeavors such as sports and recreation. He will also have better control and timing with his arms and will be able to enjoy ball activities. He will likely have exposure to computers and other technology. House Model on the next page.

Middle Childhood: 9 to 12 Years

At this stage, your child will be continuing to refine the daily living skills that require more dexterity. He probably will also be able to do things faster. Until this stage, the fine motor skills such as printing and fastening buttons and zippers on clothing still required a lot of concentration, and thus were done slowly. Although your child may still have difficulty with tying shoelaces, buttoning his cuffs, and other such tasks, he will probably

5 to 8 Years House Model

Leisure
Colors pictures;
Plays video games;
Sports activities (e.g.,
swimming, ball, etc.)

Household
Helps with household
tasks: clearing table,
dusting, sweeping

Self-Help
Uses fork/spoon well;
Pours own drink;
Grooming: starts to brush
hair/teeth;
Undresses/dresses self
with some help;
Starts to fasten
buttons/zippers

Visual Motor
Starts to form letters and
simple pictures;
Cuts lines, tries corners;
Uses glue;
Tripod grasp of pencil;
Prints most or all letters

Dexterity
Opens containers;
Can show individual fingers in turn;
Turns doorknobs;
Releases accurately;
Plays with manipulatives (e.g., Duplo, Lego);
Taps, drags in iPad games

Stability
Throws/catches a ball;
Opens and holds doors;
Turns skipping rope;
Sweeps floor

Bilateral Coordination
Folds things
(paper, towels);
Dries dishes;
Strings beads;
Sticker books;
Hand dominance evident

Sensation
Uses a backpack;
Uses a computer mouse;
Continues to enjoy
sensory play

be able to dress himself with little physical assistance. His fine motor skills may be good enough to enable him to begin to learn to type on a keyboard, to play a musical instrument, and participate in simple arts and crafts activities. Computers, smartphones, and other technology often become important to augment verbal, signed, or written communication. House Model on the next page.

9 to 12 Years House Model

Leisure
Individual/team sports;
Develops hobbies;
Arts activities (e.g., dance,
music, crafts, etc.);
Puts on own music, DVDs

Household
Prepares simple foods
(e.g., toast with butter);
Uses knife to cut;
Manages some simple
household tasks

Self-Help
Fastens buttons/zippers;
Takes responsibility for
some grooming (e.g., hair,
teeth, bathing)

Visual Motor
Prints or uses computer
for written
communication;
Uses scissors;
Dynamic tripod grasp

Dexterity
Opens packages;
Performs functions on iPad, computer;
Flips pages of books;
Manages vending/candy machines

Stability
Uses arms for strength
(swinging from bars,
gymnastics, lifting and
carrying, shoveling snow)

**Bilateral
Coordination**
Ties a knot;
Shuffles and deals cards;
Uses stencils, sticker books;
Folds paper

Sensation
Plays computer/
video games;
Can put on gloves;
Washes own hair;
Finds things in
school desk

Teen & Adult Years: 13 Years to Adulthood

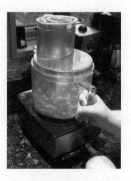

During the teen years, children with Down syndrome expand the fine motor skills learned in childhood to broader environments. By adolescence, hand movements for particular routine activities may have become more automatic, requiring less effort and concentration. Your child will generalize his fine motor abilities to all his classes at school, to his social environments, in recreation and leisure activities, and possibly to volunteer work and paid employment, which continues in adulthood. House Model below.

13 Years to Adulthood House Model

Independent Living Skills
Does volunteer/paid work;
Learns to bake and cook;
Manages self-care in different environments;
Uses machines: lawn mower, food processor, vacuum, etc.

Leisure
Manages pet care;
Initiates own hobbies;
Organizes CD's and/or
MP3 player

Household
Peels and chops
vegetables;
Makes own lunch;
Makes bed;
Does laundry

Self-Help
Uses hair dryer;
Nail care;
Shaves (with supervision);
Menstrual care

Visual Motor
May learn cursive writing;
Develops a "signature";
Uses computers

Dexterity
Opens combination lock;
Uses a pay/cell phone;
Puts notes in binder/Duo-tang;
Manages change in wallet/pocket

Stability
Carries tray of food in
cafeteria;
Carries books in busy
hallway

**Bilateral
Coordination**
Ties shoelaces;
Uses can opener;
Tears off bus tickets

Sensation
Finds items on top shelf
of locker;
Finds necessary items
in locker in busy hallway

Conclusion

Here are the main points to remember about the overall development of your child's fine motor skills:

1. **The foundation skills, or "building blocks," are very important for the development of what we think of as "fine motor skills."** Your child needs to hold his body and arms stable when using both hands together and use the "feel" of the movement to guide him when he attempts activities such as stacking blocks, stringing beads, printing, or tying shoelaces.

2. **Control of movement progresses in a proximal to distal fashion (shoulders-elbows-wrists-hands).**

3. **Children develop dexterity through play and daily activities such as eating and dressing.**

4. **All children build on previously learned skills and abilities as they learn to do more complicated fine motor tasks.** That is why a strong foundation (i.e., stability, bilateral coordination, and sensation) helps our children to move on to learn the daily living skills of self-help, school, household, and leisure activities.

5. **Our children will best learn fine motor skills (and other skills) through activities that are meaningful to them.** For example, practicing putting clothes pins (clothes pegs) on the rim of a container might not be meaningful and motivating for your child, but using clothespins to hang up his bathing suit after swimming may be.

6. **Adapt the environment to enable success in fine motor and daily living skills.**

AGES & STAGES
A Summary of Fine Motor Development

In summary, here are some of the main points to keep in mind for each stage of your child's fine motor development. Some of the things listed will be *emerging* at the end of the stage; they may not be consistent yet. For example, a child just turned two may not be isolating his index finger to point yet, but he may be pointing with his whole hand or thumb.

Infancy to 2 Years
- Encourage your baby to weight bear on his arms and hands (i.e., pushing himself up with his hands when on his tummy).
- Encourage your baby to reach up with his hands when he is on his back.
- Provide supportive sitting positions so your baby can begin to develop accurate reaching and eye-hand coordination.
- Provide toys that your baby can easily grasp with both hands, pass from hand to hand, and put in his mouth.
- Show your child how to take things out and put them into containers.
- Provide activity boxes and cause-effect toys.
- Encourage your child to point at pictures in books and to objects and to poke his fingers into holes.
- Encourage finger feeding, and introduce a child's spoon and small cup.
- Provide sensory play experiences.
- When your child is grasping something and banging it, make sure his thumb is around the toy, not tucked into his palm.
- Play simple social games (e.g., peek-a-boo), sing simple songs with actions.

2 to 4 Years
- Provide toys that come apart and fit back together.
- Provide toys that have parts that go into holes, slots, and spaces (e.g., puzzles and shape sorters).
- Hold up small items (such as bits of food) for your child to attempt to grasp with his index finger and thumb (pincer grasp).
- Use block and large pegboard activities to encourage the thumb and fingers to pick up in a tripod grasp and to let go more precisely (e.g., pegs into holes, stacking blocks).
- Provide opportunities for sensory play (water, sand, paint, etc.).

- Introduce markers, crayons, etc. and encourage your child's expression on paper.
- Introduce scissors and let your child experiment with them. Demonstrate the correct grasp, but your child may not be ready to hold them this way yet.
- Use daily activities that encourage your child to hold things in his palm (e.g., pouring soap, shampoo, or vitamins into his palm).
- Provide manipulative toys (e.g., Duplo, Tinker Toys).
- Encourage your child to participate as much as possible in dressing and toileting.
- Teach your child how to scoop with a spoon, drink from a cup, and place the cup down after drinking.
- Do pouring activities in the bathtub or sink or with dry sensory materials.
- Do action songs and rhymes together.
- Provide activities with push-pull actions of the arms (e.g., climbing, using push toys).

5 to 8 Years

- Sing songs that have individual finger movements and actions (e.g., "Eensy Weensy Spider").
- Encourage your child to position a marker/pencil in a tripod grasp in his hand.
- Do some drawing, preprinting, and, when ready, printing activities at various surfaces (easel or table).
- Provide simple matching, dot-to-dot, maze, and coloring activities.
- Do pouring activities with small jugs of liquid or dry ingredients.
- Encourage your child to do most of his dressing and undressing, including attempting fastenings such as zippers and buttons.
- Encourage your child to pick up and release small items into a precise spot (e.g., coins into a piggy bank).
- Encourage your child to hold scissors with his hand in mid-position with his thumb up, and to snip, cut across a strip, etc.
- Provide opportunities for strengthening pincer grasp (e.g., clothespins, play dough activities).
- Provide bilateral hand activities and manipulative toys (e.g., threading beads, building with Duplo and Lego).
- Introduce printing activities on lines and in workbooks as he is ready.
- Encourage your child to begin to participate in household activities, such as folding laundry, setting the table, sweeping, etc.
- Encourage your child to cut his own food and pour his own drink.

9 to 12 Years

- Encourage your child to more actively participate in household chores (e.g., sweeping and vacuuming, folding laundry, etc.).
- Provide bilateral hand activities that require small movements of the fingers and wrists (e.g., sticker books, stencils, folding paper, as in making a paper airplane).
- Provide opportunities for individual finger movement, such as with a computer or tablet keyboard, a music keyboard, or recorder.
- Encourage your child to hold a fork in a mature grasp and to cut and spread with a knife.
- Give him opportunities to open packages and containers.
- Encourage your child to pick up small items one at a time and store them in his palm.
- Encourage strength and control of pincer grasp with activities such as using thumbtacks and large paper clips.
- Help him practice choosing his own clothes to wear and fastening his own zippers and buttons. Encourage him to dress himself.
- Encourage your child to manage some of his grooming, such as hair care, washing himself, etc.
- Support him in his printing efforts, and perhaps introduce pre-writing and cursive writing activities, if appropriate.
- Help your child develop rewarding leisure-time activities.
- Play games that involve finger movement and control, such as Ker-Plunk, Barrel of Monkeys, Jenga, card games, etc.

13 Years to Adulthood

- Encourage your child in regular physical activity and leisure activities.
- Maintain his upper body strength through activities such as swimming, basketball, baseball, gardening, etc.
- Encourage him to develop a signature.
- Encourage computer and tablet keyboard use.
- Encourage him to choose his own clothing and to dress independently.
- Encourage him to manage his self-care and grooming independently.
- Teach aspects of adolescent self-care (such as shaving, menstrual care) by modeling, gradually reducing assistance as appropriate.
- Encourage continued development of dexterity with speed and control of fine movements in activities he enjoys (e.g., cooking, sewing, building models, etc.).
- Encourage using fine motor skills for learning community living skills, such as using a computer to find a library book, using a bank machine, etc.

Early Movement in Babies with Down Syndrome

In the early months, development of fine and gross motor skills goes hand in hand. With each new gross motor skill learned, your baby is also preparing her arms and hands for the many hand functions she will have to perform as she matures. She is building stability and sensory awareness in her arms and hands and learning to use both arms to help her move around on the floor. She is building her foundations for fine motor skills: *stability, bilateral coordination,* and *sensation.*

Stability	**Bilateral Coordination**	**Sensation**
Gaining control of her movement; Holding herself upright; Uses arms for support and to reach	Using both hands and both sides of her body for movement and play	Learning to respond to what she feels and to the sensation of changing her body position

This chapter will describe how your baby is preparing for fine motor skills while she is mastering gross motor milestones. For detailed descriptions of how to help your child achieve gross motor skills, refer to *Gross Motor Skills in Children with Down Syndrome* (Patricia C. Winders, Woodbine House, 2014).

How Can I Help My Baby Develop Early Arm Movements?

Described below are the early gross motor milestones and their relationship to later fine motor development. Suggestions are given to help your baby and young child with Down syndrome develop and coordinate arm movements in various positions. The focus of fine motor development during the early milestones is on:

1. Strength: using the arms to hold, position, and move the body in and out of various positions
2. Reach: Using the arms and hands to reach and grasp, which positions the hands for function

Lying on Back and Side
Lifting Arms When on Back

Lifting arms and feet when on her back prepares your baby for accurately placing and holding her arms within her visual field, the beginnings of eye-hand coordination. Early on, this will simply be too difficult for your baby, because of low muscle tone and poor stability in the shoulders. These are the steps in learning to lift her arms up and hold them there:

1. lying in side lying, bringing her hands up in front of her face;
2. sitting in a supportive, semi-reclined infant seat, bringing her hands together in the center;
3. swiping at toys in side lying and in an infant seat;
4. reaching up for faces and to swipe at toys in back lying, with support under the shoulders;
5. reaching out and grasping toys in side lying and in an infant seat;
6. reaching up and grasping suspended toys in back lying;
7. holding and playing with a toy, such as a rattle, in an infant seat;
8. holding and playing with a toy, such as a rattle, in back lying.

Side Lying: In this position your baby will be able to bring her hands together and look at them without having to work against gravity. The goal is to have hands together in side lying, with feet also coming forward, to activate tummy muscles. If she arches her back in this position, try to tuck her chin towards her chest, and bring her legs forward, to activate the muscles on the front of her body.

Semi-Reclined: In an infant seat (including a car seat), your baby can begin to develop arm strength against gravity in a semi-reclined position, which is easier than lifting her arms when on her back. Her chin should be lightly tucked to activate muscles in the front of the neck and shoulder area.

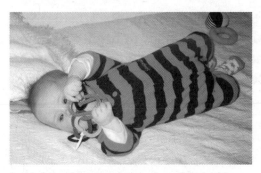

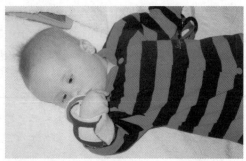

In side lying, this young baby can easily bring his hands together to hold toys where he can see them and bring them to his mouth.

Soft Velcro wrist toys help an infant become aware of his hands. The toy can also be placed around his ankle.

Back Lying with Support: If your baby attempts to lift her arms when she is on her back, but can't lift them up high enough to be able to see them, place small rolls (towels or baby blankets), or a cloth infant car seat insert under her shoulders. This also helps her to tuck her chin. At first you may need to place a soft toy right on her chest, as this may be as far as she can reach. This helps her lift her hands up where she can see them. Looking at her hands is very important at this stage. As her shoulders and arms get stronger, she can progress to reaching for overhead toys.

Babies also like to lift their feet up into the air when on their backs, reaching out for their toes with their hands. Often, a baby with Down syndrome will attempt to grasp her feet by bending her knees outward, and bringing her feet together. If she grasps her feet in this way, she isn't using her tummy muscles to pull her legs up. She needs your help initially to hold her knees in line with her hips, so she can learn to use her tummy muscles to lift her legs. Developing strength in her tummy muscles is important for fine motor skills because these muscles help the baby have a stable base from which to move her arms and hands.

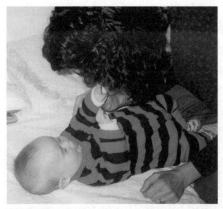

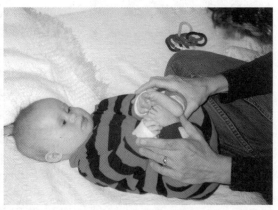

Your baby will enjoy reaching up to touch your face and hair.

Help your baby to reach up and grasp his or her toes.

Fine Motor Skills in Side Lying, Semi-Reclined, and Back Lying: Side lying, semi-reclined, and back lying are good positions to begin fine motor skill development in the first few months of life. The baby is comfortable in these positions, and can easily hold her head in the center (midline), with-

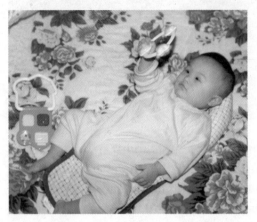

out having to work hard to hold her head up. In side lying she can easily bring her hands up in front of her face where she can see them. Sitting in an infant seat and back lying are natural positions for face-to-face interaction with parents, siblings, etc. Babies are instinctively interested in faces, and quite early on learn to discriminate features of familiar faces and voices. Playing with your baby in this position will encourage her to reach up to your face and hair. Your

A car seat head support can help position the baby's head and shoulders to enable her to lift her arms.

positive response will lead her to do this again and again. This is the first step in learning to reach out, touch, and grasp something she wants. It will help her develop early control of her arm and hand movements.

Initially, any reaching out your baby does is with large swiping movements that are not very accurate. At this stage, suspended overhead toys are helpful, as your baby can reach up, swipe at the dangling toy, watch it spin and move, and listen to the noise it makes. Some baby activity gyms have toys along the side bars that are useful when the baby is playing in side lying.

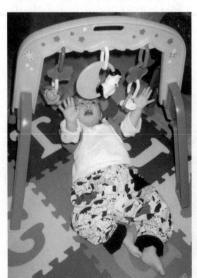

Weighted toys that make a noise but don't roll away when the baby moves them, such as the vintage Fisher-Price Roly Poly Chime Ball or the Happy Apple, or the newer Fisher-Price Crawl Along Snail, can be positioned within reach when your baby is in side lying. She is reinforced for her efforts to reach out by the noise and movement of the toy.

You can also encourage your baby to lift and move her hands in the air by putting a soft wrist rattle on her arm. These soft toys will not hurt her if she drops her arm to her face. They can also be placed around your baby's ankle, if you are at the stage of encouraging her to lift and play with her feet.

Toys suspended overhead can help motivate a baby to lift his arms.

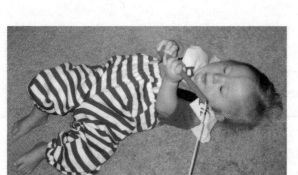

This baby can reach up and hold both arms up to play. His hands are together in midline where he can easily see them.

As your baby's arm movements become more accurate, she will be able to bring her hand directly to the toy without the large sweeping arm movements of the first few months of life. At this stage, you can progress to toys that can easily be grasped. These include rings or toys that have handles, such as rattles. Place the toy on the floor if your baby is in side lying, or hold it above her if she is in an infant seat or lying on her back. Now she will be able to grasp the overhead play gym rather than simply swiping at it; if she has difficulty grasping it because it moves, hold it steady for her.

Lying on Stomach
Propping Up on Arms When on Tummy

Propping up on her arms when on her tummy (prone) helps your baby develop stability and strength in her shoulder, arm, and neck muscles. It also prepares your baby's shoulder muscles for accurate reaching and the stability to hold her arms steady while performing precise hand movements. Some babies with Down syndrome resist being on their tummies. It is worthwhile to persist with this position and experiment with various motivators, as developing arm strength in this position is important for both future gross motor milestones and fine motor skill development.

This is the progression of fine motor development in the propped position, when your baby is on her stomach:

1. lifting her head with support on elbows;
2. lifting her head and chest with support on elbows;
3. lifting her head and chest with support on hands;
4. reaching forward with one hand, with support on other elbow;
5. reaching forward with one hand, with support on other hand;
6. reaching up with one hand, with support on other hand;
7. pivoting in a circle, using arms to move.

At first (about two or three months of age), your baby will use her neck and shoulder muscles to lift and hold her head up. Help her position her arms with her elbows directly under her shoulders or slightly forward, so that she is taking weight through her shoulders and forearms. This will help her lift her head up. Keeping the arms slightly forward helps to activate a balance of muscles between the front and back of the body.

At this stage, activity quilts can be fun. These baby quilts have small mirrors, squeeze toys, animal faces, etc., sewn right into them. Your baby will be motivated to prop herself up on her arms to see in the mirror or to reach for the squeeze toys. Eventually, she will be able to push right up, supporting herself on her hands. This position is excellent for developing strength in the neck, shoulders, arms, wrists, and hands.

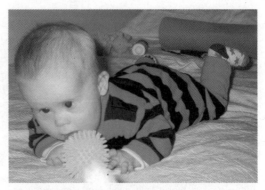

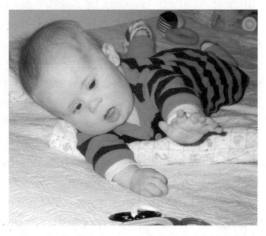

This baby can hold his head up briefly and is beginning to take weight through his forearms. He can move one hand forward on the surface to reach for the toy.

A baby with Down syndrome may "hyperextend" her neck when on her stomach. She literally pulls her head back and rests it on her upper back, due to weakness in the neck muscles. If she continues to do this, she will not develop the strength in her neck muscles necessary for holding her head up in other positions, such as sitting. If your baby hyperextends her head, try supporting her elbows and shoulders with your hands, and lowering anything that she is looking at (including yourself!). Continue to work on head control when holding her upright on your shoulder and when on your lap. (See *Gross Motor Skills in Children with Down Syndrome,* by Patricia Winders.)

With a small roll under his chest, he can lift his arm up off the surface to reach. He may roll onto his side, but will get better control of his head position and weight shifting as he gets strong in this position.

Sometimes therapists use a small wedge, roll, or rolled-up towel under the baby's chest to help position her arms for propping. Other tummy-play products are commercially available, such as Tumzee and

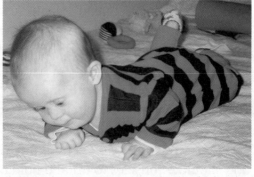

The baby then begins to try to push up on his hands.

the Infantino tummy time activity mat. These items can initially help your baby experience the position, but should be discontinued as soon as she can hold herself up to play on her tummy on her own.

Reaching and Pivoting When Propping on Arms: When your baby can hold herself in a propped position briefly, either on elbows or hands, she is ready to begin reaching out with one hand. In order to do this, she must shift her body weight over to one arm, while reaching forward for a toy with the other hand. When first learning to do this, your baby might shift her weight too far and consequently roll over. For some babies, this may be the way they learn to roll from stomach to back.

It is important for your baby to learn how to move her weight over to one side in order to learn how to creep and crawl. When she shifts her weight to one side, she increases the stability and strength on that side. She should take turns shifting weight to either side and reaching with both hands. First she will reach forward for a toy on the floor. Because she is working so hard to hold herself up while moving her arm forward, she will need a toy that she can swipe at, or a toy that can be easily grasped (such as the Skwish rattle). She may grasp it and pull it in toward her body so she can put it in her mouth. Be sure to use soft toys that will not hurt her as she pulls them in toward her face.

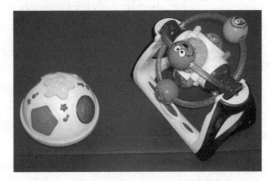

Examples of toys that respond to touch with lights and music: motivating for a baby beginning to reach out when on her stomach.

As she gets stronger in the propped position, she will be able to lift one arm right up off the floor to reach a toy you are holding up for her. At first she will immediately drop her arm back down to the floor, but as she develops more strength, she will be able to hold her arm up to shake or bang the toy. If your baby always falls over onto her side when trying to reach in this position, it may be because she is moving her head too far over to that side as well. She has to learn to shift her weight onto one arm while holding her head steady in the center. This is how you can help her learn to support her weight on one arm while reaching with the other:

1. If you would like her to reach with her right hand, place your hand firmly over her left hip to help her shift her weight over to the left side of her body.
2. With your other hand, support her left shoulder so she holds herself up through her arm without rolling to the left. This will also help her keep her head upright.
3. If necessary, prompt her to reach for the toy with her right hand.

When your baby has learned to reach up with one hand, she will be ready to pivot around on her stomach. To pivot, your baby turns to one side, where a toy is positioned, and uses her arms to move herself around in a circle to reach the toy. To do this, she must shift her weight alternately from one arm to the other, and pull her body around, using mainly the movements of her arms. Pivoting helps to develop strength in your baby's shoulders and arms.

Commando Crawling: As the baby learns to shift her weight from one side to the other, she can learn to use arm strength to pull herself forward on the floor, using alternating elbow and forearm. She coordinates this with her leg movements.

Rolling Over

Rolling from stomach to back usually develops before pivoting. Rolling over prepares your baby for using one arm differently from the other by changing her center of gravity from one side to the other. All of these activities that involve shifting weight from one arm to the other are important in helping your baby develop the adjustments in her body and arms necessary for balance later on. Body and shoulder adjustments are also very important during the school years, in visual motor activities such as cutting, as your child guides her hands through complex movements.

Rolling from stomach to back usually develops before rolling from back to stomach, often when the baby leans over while propping on her stomach. When rolling from her back to her stomach, your baby has to be much more active with her movements, lifting her legs to initiate the roll, and lifting her arm up and over to the other side.

Sitting
Supported Sitting

Babies with Down syndrome usually take a long time to learn to sit independently because of hypotonia and shorter arm length. A delay in independent floor sitting should not hold your baby back from playing and using her hands while sitting, however. At this stage of development, babies are learning how to pick up and let go of toys of various sizes and shapes. If your baby spends part of her day in a well-supported sitting position, she will be able to begin developing more controlled grasp and release patterns for play. Give her opportunities to play while sitting upright in a highchair, floor sitter, or similar supportive seat.

Highchairs are usually designed with head and side support, safety straps, and a wrap-around tray. Sitting in a highchair for some play activities gives your baby a chance to move her arms, hands, and fingers more freely than she can on the floor. Because she has good support from the highchair, she can focus on using her hands to learn and discover things and doesn't have to worry about falling over. This positioning helps with sitting balance and

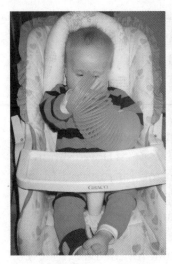

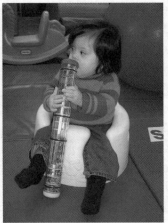

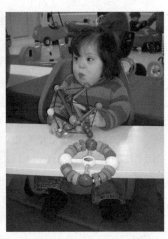

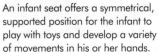

An infant seat offers a symmetrical, supported position for the infant to play with toys and develop a variety of movements in his or her hands.

A "Bumbo seat" provides support for the baby who is not yet able to use both hands freely in play when sitting on the floor. The Flip 'n Sit is another example of a floor seat; it can also be used on a chair. Here, a wooden bench is used as a play surface.

keeping hands in the center (midline), so your child can easily see and play using both hands. If your baby needs more support than the high chair offers, you can use small rolled-up towels on either side, or a piece of firm foam behind her back. Use a piece of non-slip matting on the seat to prevent your baby from sliding forward.

You will be able to offer your baby more challenging fine motor toys when she is sitting in the highchair than when she is on the floor. For example, she will likely be better able to grasp and move the knobs and buttons on a busy box when she is sitting in the highchair than when she is sitting on the floor.

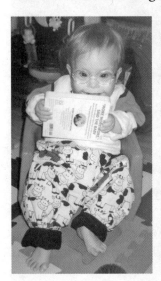

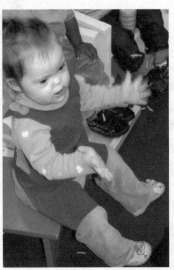

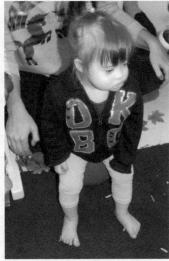

Left, sitting on a stool or booster seat helps the child learn to take weight through his or her legs and feet, in preparation for standing. Other seating options include a bench or small ball, as these children are sitting on during circle time at preschool.

Once your baby has developed head and trunk control, seats with support for the pelvis and legs, such as the "Bumbo Babysitter" seat and tray, Ingenuity baby seat with tray, and the "Flip 'n Sit" seat, can be used. (See Resources section for availability.)

Floor Sitting

Most babies use their hands on the floor to prop themselves up when they are first learning to sit. This is a difficult position for babies with Down syndrome because their arms are shorter and they have to lean too far forward to prop themselves. If your baby tries to sit propping on her arms, she may rest her head back on her upper back, which is not a position you want to encourage. Give her some support in front to rest her arms on, so she can sit up straight while propping herself. I like to use a cardboard box (with a cutout for the baby's legs) or a bench or firm cushion, upon which toys can be placed. Your baby may also need some support behind her, so she doesn't fall backward. A firm sofa cushion, mother's nursing cushion, or similar support behind the hips can be used.

Your baby will need the support of your hands, or supportive cushions, pillows, or rolls around her hips and lower back when sitting on the floor until she develops enough control of her tummy and back muscles to sit up on her own. With help and practice, your baby will gradually develop the strength in these muscles to be able to sit independently.

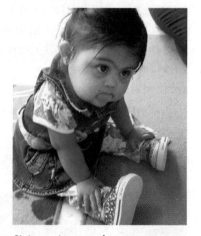

Sitting, using arms for support.

These are the steps in fine motor development in floor sitting:

1. The baby sits with arms supported on a box or cushion, looking at a toy.
2. One arm props on a box or cushion for support in sitting, while the other hand holds a toy.
3. The toy is still supported on a box or cushion, but the baby can now use both hands to play.
4. The baby can play with a toy using both hands without front support.
5. The baby can reach out and take a toy from you.
6. The baby can reach forward to pick up a toy from the floor and sit back up.
7. The baby can reach to the side to pick up a toy and sit back up.
8. The baby can shake, bang, and throw toys in sitting and maintain balance.
9. The baby can turn to reach a toy behind her, leaning on one hand and reaching with the other, and then sitting back up.

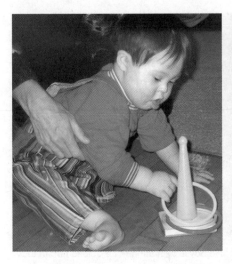
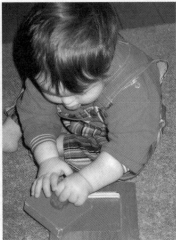

This baby uses one hand for balance in floor sitting. He can manage a one-handed activity, but would have more success with two-handed activities like this puzzle seated in a highchair or at a table.

As your baby gains better control of her back and tummy muscles to maintain her balance in sitting, her arms become freer to move.

Once they have learned to sit independently, babies with Down syndrome often prefer to sit on the floor with their legs in a "frog-legged" or "ring" position: spread wide at the hips, knees out, feet together. Alternately, they may sit with legs out stiffly straight and knees locked. It is important that your baby also experience sitting with her knees in line with her hips and her feet flat on the floor. A booster seat on the floor provides some back and side support, while encouraging weight bearing through the feet. Similarly, a small stool or bench encourages her to sit with her feet flat on the floor. This helps her develop better use of all her leg muscles, and allows her to learn to balance using her tummy and back muscles.

Practicing balance, reaching, and turning in different sitting positions will help your child develop body and arm stability, strength, and control for fine motor skills. The muscles of the back, tummy, and neck provide the base that the arms need in order to move and direct the hands into position. When she is ready, challenge your child to reach in different directions for toys, both in floor sitting and on a bench or stool. By doing this she learns to control the movement of her body while accurately reaching out with her arms.

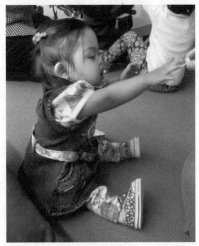

Moving into and out of Sitting

Young children with Down syndrome often move their whole body rather than

This child maintains her balance while reaching forward. As her sitting balance develops, she will be able to reach to the side and back, shifting her weight through her base of support as she does so.

turning (rotating) part of their body. For example, rather than turning to one side to lower down to the floor or to begin crawling from floor sitting, your baby may do the "splits," lower her upper body down to the floor, and then swing her legs back behind her. Although effective (she gets down!), she is avoiding challenging her balance and isn't turning her body. It is better to help her place one arm down to the side while turning herself to that side. Again, this helps strengthen the shoulder muscles.

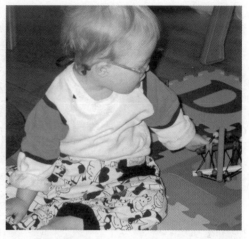

This little boy is beginning to be able to turn to the side in sitting to reach for a toy. He is reaching for a Skwish rattle, which is a wonderful toy for babies: easy to grasp, colorful, with bells.

Pushing Up into a Crawling Position (Hands and Knees)

The terms *creeping* and *crawling* may refer to different movement patterns, depending on where you live, and which type of developmental or medical specialist you are speaking to. The "hands and knees" position is called *quadruped*, or *four-point*. Moving forward with alternate movements of arms and legs from the four-point position (stomach up off the floor) will be referred to as crawling in this book, as this is the commonly understood meaning of the word.

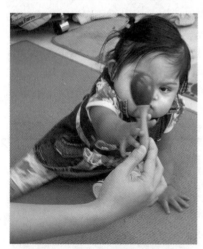

This child is transitioning out of sitting into hands and knees while reaching.

Before crawling, your baby will try to move herself with her stomach down on the floor by pushing with her arms and legs to one side (pivoting in a circle), and pulling herself forward with her elbows (commando crawling).

On hands and knees, the baby prepares her hands for fine movements by rocking backward and forward and side to side. Leaning on their hands and rocking helps babies develop the different muscles in their hands and strengthens their shoulders and arms. It also helps to develop the arches of the hands, which we will talk about in more detail in Chapter 8.

Again, low muscle tone and shorter arms will make it harder for your baby to assume and hold this position at first. A firm cushion under her hands will help initially. Once she is able to hold herself in this position, you may be able to encourage rocking back and forth by singing or playing music. Her hands should be open; her fists shouldn't be clenched.

These are the steps in fine motor development in the hands and knees position:

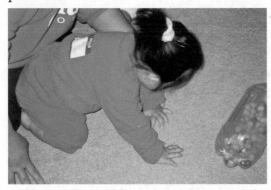

1. The baby supports herself on hands and knees, with someone supporting her at her hips.
2. The baby holds herself on hands and knees, with a cushion under her hands.
3. The baby holds herself on hands and knees without a cushion.
4. The baby rocks forward and backward and side to side on her hands and knees.
5. The baby reaches out with one hand for a toy, holding the hands-and-knees position.

A little support at the hips helps this child hold herself in the hands-and-knees position (quadruped). She will progress to holding this position independently and then to lifting one hand to reach for a toy, in preparation for pulling to stand.

6. The baby moves into hands and knees from sitting and then moves back into sitting by turning to one side.
7. The baby can shift weight and coordinate movements to crawl. It is common for babies with Down syndrome to develop alternate ways to move themselves forward, such as thrusting themselves forward with both arms at once.

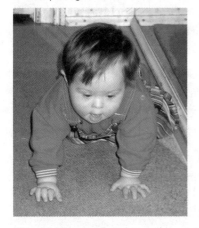

This child has developed enough stability to lift his hands to crawl

The progression of use of the hands is essentially the same as in the propped position. First the baby must learn to hold the position, then to assume and hold the position, and then to shift her weight to one side so she can reach with the other hand for a toy. This weight shifting will eventually help her learn to crawl forward on hands and knees.

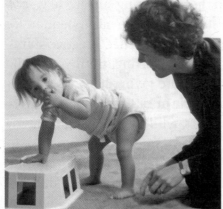

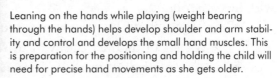

Leaning on the hands while playing (weight bearing through the hands) helps develop shoulder and arm stability and control and develops the small hand muscles. This is preparation for the positioning and holding the child will need for precise hand movements as she gets older.

Pulling to Stand and Standing

Your baby develops stability and strength in her shoulder muscles as she uses her arms to pull herself up to standing. She uses a power grasp in her hands to hold onto an edge as she pulls herself up. To help her learn to stand, try the following:

1. Start by having her sit on a stool or in a booster seat, with her feet firmly on the floor.
2. Give her a firm surface to pull up on, such as the edge of a coffee table, a chair, a stair banister, or your hands.
3. When she can pull herself up from a stool, progress to having her start in the kneeling position, bringing one foot forward first, then the other, as she rises.

Fine Motor Development in Standing: Your child can practice fine motor skills in standing with either front or back support. Standing with her back in a corner or against a wall allows her to use her arms more freely. Be aware that the level of fine motor play that she will be capable of when learning to stand will be lower than the level she can accomplish in supported sitting. For example, if she can fill and empty containers with blocks when she is in her highchair, she may be able to watch a music box or bang a xylophone when learning to stand. When she is learning to stand, she will primarily be using her hands for balance, not for fine motor skill development.

With front support, she will need to hold on to the table edge or rail with both hands initially, and thus her hands will not be free for play. As she gets stronger and develops better control in standing, she will be able to lift one hand to play while supporting herself with her other hand. Still holding herself with one hand on the surface, she will next be able to reach to the side and to squat down to reach a toy on the floor. Gradually she will be able to use her hands more and more while standing, shifting her supporting hand from one side to the other and then letting go very briefly with both hands.

It is better not to let your child lean into the supporting surface (e.g., coffee table) with her chest in order to play in standing. If she has to lean in for chest support, the activity is probably still too difficult for her. Practice standing with both hands supporting, then one hand supporting, until your child has good standing balance in these positions, before giving her toys that require two hands to play with. From the coffee table or rail she can progress to placing one hand on the wall or fridge for support, while reaching and playing with her other hand.

When standing with back support, your child can progress from standing in the corner or against the wall to standing with support behind her legs, as with a small chair or stool. In these positions, you can give her pro-

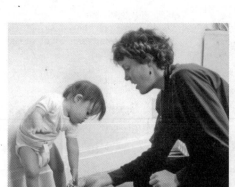

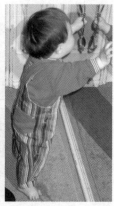

Standing against a wall in a corner or pushing against it for support helps children learn to use their arms while balancing their body in standing.

gressively more challenging reaching and play opportunities, as her balance in standing improves.

Cruising: As the child gains more stability and balance in standing, she begins to shift weight through her body, legs, and feet, allowing her to side step and cruise along furniture. She uses her arms for support on the surface as she cruises sideways.

Postural Stability Supports

Some physical and occupational therapists recommend postural support systems to help children maintain the upright positions of sitting and standing. These special garments provide biomechanical support (structural support of the muscles and bones) and sensory input and help maintain good alignment and support while the child is developing postural and movement control. In my experience, the two types of postural support systems commonly recommended are:

1. Postural support garments such as TheraTogs or SPIO
2. Kinesiotaping

Postural Support Garments: TheraTogs (www.theratogs.com) are described as orthotic garments and strapping systems that a child wears to replicate the gentle alignment guidance and postural positioning she receives during hands-on therapy. The fit and strapping are customized to each child and must be supervised by a therapist knowledgeable in its use.

In working with young children with Down syndrome, I have found that the support provided by TheraTogs can help a young child achieve and maintain upright postures, providing a more stable base from which to use her arms and hands functionally. The system can also help facilitate the functioning of the abdominal muscles. When children with Down syndrome learn to sit, they often do so with externally rotated and abducted hips, which widens the base of support and decreases the active use of trunk and hip muscles. TheraTogs can align the spine and pelvis and activate the abdominal and hip muscles, which can help children reduce their base of support.

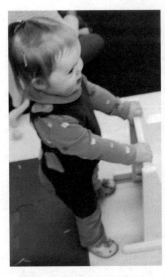
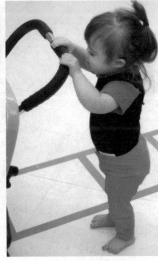

(Left) TheraTogs helps this child maintain good alignment as she is learning to stand.
(Right) This little girl is wearing a SPIO garment.

Because TheraTogs activates muscles in new ways and in new alignment, wearing them can be fatiguing for the child. Parents, caregivers, and therapists must carefully monitor the child for fatigue and adjust the wear schedule. TheraTogs can help cue the child's muscles; the child must then be given plenty of opportunity to experience the same positions without wearing the support.

SPIO is a dynamic, flexible lycra compression garment that provides deep pressure. SPIO body suits (vests, short- and long-sleeved tops, and pants) help some children control their posture and movement and may help them regulate sensory input that may otherwise be overwhelming. SPIO was specifically designed to be worn all day by children who have special needs.

Kinesiotape: Kinesiotape is a rehabilitative taping technique that has a broad range of uses. For children with Down syndrome, it can be used to reeducate the dynamic balance of muscle use while providing support and stability to muscles and joints. Depending on how it is applied, kinesiotape can help muscles activate or can help relax overworked, tight muscles. I have seen it used successfully for activation of abdominal muscles, and to achieve balanced muscle activation during specific movement patterns. For example, kinesiotape can be applied to support an unstable thumb joint, thus helping the child achieve a pincer grasp. It must be applied by a therapist trained in kinesiotape application.

Conclusion

In the first stages of development, the focus is on the achievement of gross motor skills. This chapter has described how your baby will use her arms and hands during gross motor development and how these early fine motor skills relate to the more precise hand movements she will develop in the next stages. While your baby is working on gross motor milestones, she will also be getting ready to develop aspects of dexterity, such as picking objects up and letting them go, pointing, and passing things from hand to hand. Whatever your child's stage of gross motor development, you would therefore benefit from reading the following chapters.

Grandma's and Grandpa's List

Many of us are fortunate enough to have parents who ask for suggestions of what to buy our children for their birthdays and other special occasions. Here are a few suggestions of toys and equipment that help fine motor development in approximately the first two years of your baby's life. Bear in mind that although I may give an example of the type of toy, there are often several other brands of the same type of toy that would work just as well.

- Baby play activity gym (sometimes called infant development systems, or play zones)
- Weighted or suction cup toys for baby to swipe at
- Activity center/board/table
- Activity quilt
- Infant seat (e.g., Bumbo, Ingenuity)
- Tummy play support (e.g., Tumzee; Infantino Tummy Time Activity Mat)
- Chair support (tie-around support to use in a regular chair, if a highchair is not available)
- Head hugger (support for head in car or infant seat)
- Sleep time support pillow (to support neck in car seat)
- Highchair (with wrap-around tray and contoured sides); booster seat
- Soft wrist, ankle, and foot rattle sets
- Rattles and squeeze toys that are easy to grasp
- Chewing toys/teething rings
- Touch and feel books; board books; Taggies books
- Skwish rattle; Skwish Stix sensory toy with suction cup
- Loopy links
- Baby mirror
- Soft stuffed animals
- Suction toys (for standing up on the highchair tray)

5

The First Building Block:
Stability

At seven and a half, Sarah could pull a toboggan up a hill. She could push another child on a swing and swing from her arms across a row of monkey bars. She had developed reasonably good stability in her body and shoulders to do these things. But when she was printing, the letters were usually so light you could hardly see them. She had not yet developed enough consistent stability and strength in her hands. I say consistent, because she could briefly use enough strength to print darker, but couldn't maintain it when she was concentrating so hard on the formation of the letters.

Consistent stability is difficult for many children with Down syndrome. By "consistent stability," I mean the ability to maintain the muscular contraction around a joint to hold it in a certain position. Low muscle tone makes it more difficult to hold a consistent degree of muscle contraction over a period of time. You may find that your child can seem very strong when he wants to be. Perhaps when he gets hold of a candy bar in the grocery store, you may find it almost impossible to release his tightly clenched fingers. This, however, is different from the postural control and balance of muscle contraction needed by the same child to hold his arms and wrist steady while building a block tower. It is also different from the contraction needed by a baby to prop himself up on his arms and play in that position for several minutes. The stability that is often challenging for our children is not to intermittently tighten the muscles briefly and then release, but to hold and position themselves most efficiently for the activity.

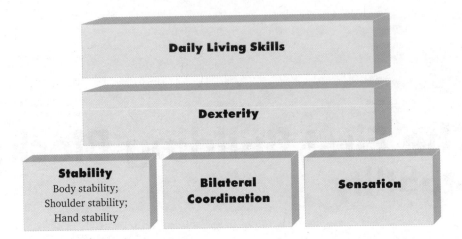

Our children need to develop three main types of stability:

1. **Body stability:** Body stability allows the child to move his arms freely while maintaining the body in a secure, balanced position.

2. **Shoulder stability:** Shoulder stability allows the child to move his lower arms and hands freely while his shoulders position his arms (such as when cutting). It also enables the arms to support the weight of the body (as when doing a push-up), and to keep the arms and hands steady when the body is moving (such as when carrying a tray of food in the cafeteria).

3. **Hand stability:** When the child is developing the ability to perform more difficult fine motor skills, such as printing, he needs to learn to use one part of his hand for stability and the other part for movement. Usually the outer edge of the hand (the baby finger side) is steady while the thumb, index, and middle fingers manipulate the object. This type of stability will be discussed in Chapter 8.

These types of stability are interconnected. We activate all types of stability when we perform activities such as:

- pushing open a door while walking through it and
- walking while holding something steady with both hands, such as a tray of drinks.

How Can I Help My Child Develop Stability?

When your child is still at the pre-walking stage, using the positions and adaptations described in Chapter 4 will help develop the early stability in the body and shoulders that he needs. Even after your child has learned to stand and walk alone, he will continue to improve his stability for many years. This section includes some activities that will help your child practice the stability that will provide him with a good "building block" for fine motor skills.

1. Body Stability
Pushing/Pulling Activities

This category includes actions that require maintaining body balance and stability while the arms are exerting force, either pushing away from the body or pulling toward the body.

Activity Walkers and Push Toys

Your child can use push toys both to help him maintain balance while walking and to help him develop body stability. Most toddlers and young children love to play with a variety of push toys. The progression will be as follows:

1. A push toy of suitable height and weight can assist your child in learning to walk. The handle should be approximately at elbow height or slightly higher. The toy should be stable enough not to topple if your child leans on it. There are many commercially available early walking/push toys such as the Fisher-Price Stride-to-Ride Dino and Fisher-Price Activity Walker. Try the toy with your child before purchasing it, if possible, to check the height and weight.

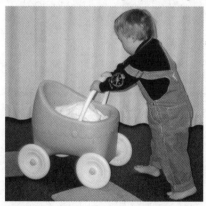

2. Pushing a light wheeled toy, such as the Fisher-Price Popper, while standing or walking helps your child learn to balance while moving his arms freely. These long-handled toys are usually pushed with one hand while the child stands or walks. An example of a lightweight push toy that needs to be pushed with both hands is a toy lawn mower. As these toys are lightweight, they can be used once your child can stand and walk independently, without needing support.

Walking while pushing toys develops body & shoulder stability, as well as hand strength.

3. Initially, your child will push the toy in a straight line. Next he will learn how to back up and pull the toy when he gets stuck.

4. As your child's balance in walking improves, he will be able to steer the walk toy to change direction and go around corners. He will learn to initiate this movement from his shoulders and to

make adjustments with his arms and body as he refines his steering. This ability to make fine adjustments is important later when he is learning visual motor skills, such as tracing. Similarly, pushing and pulling a wagon applies the same stability learning.

Pushing/Pulling Open Doors

Most children go through a stage when they love to open and close cupboard doors and drawers (usually emptying the contents in the process!). This is a normal and important developmental stage, and rather than restricting all cupboards and drawers with child safety latches, assign one that is safe for your child to experiment with.

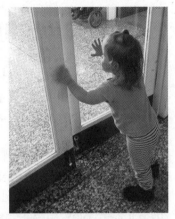

Doors at home and in the community provide opportunities for opening and for holding open the door, which improves strength and stability. Let your child do the door opening and holding when you are going into stores, etc.

Pushing open doors helps develop shoulder stability.

Pushing a Swing

Here, the force of a moving object is added, which is more challenging for a child's balance than some of the other activities above. The arms and body must absorb the force and push against it.

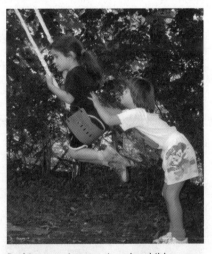

1. A good warm-up activity is to roll a large inflated exercise gym ball back and forth when standing. Your child maintains body stability and balance, and pushes the ball back to you when it rolls toward him.

2. Initially, place a doll or stuffed animal in a baby swing for your child to push.

Pushing a swing requires the child to maintain body stability while the arms move to push.

3. Progress to pushing another person. To avoid being hit, your child must be careful not to stand too close to the swing.

Digging, Shoveling, Sweeping Activities

The arms move to dig, lift, sweep, rake, etc., while the muscles of the body activate to maintain balance. These activities also develop strength in the hands. Examples of shoveling materials are sand, snow, or dry materials in a bin or container, such as dried beans, macaroni, or cornmeal.

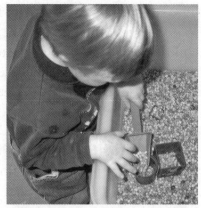

1. Begin by having your child use small shovels while sitting.
2. Progress to larger shovels that have long handles, so your child can shovel while standing.
3. Provide child-sized brooms, garden shovels, and rakes.

Shoveling develops stability and movement control in the upper arm and shoulders while also developing hand strength and wrist control.

The body and legs remain stable while the arms work together in a sideways or forward/back motion. As your child gains skill, have him try sweeping out from under furniture; this requires bending of the body and offers more of a challenge. Vacuuming offers similar opportunities to develop stability. Sweeping, vacuuming, and raking are also good bilateral coordination activities, as both arms move and apply force together.

Scarf, Streamer, Bubble Wand Play

These activities all engage the arms in large, flowing movements, while the body remains balanced and centered. Sitting or standing, your child can hold a scarf, streamer, or bubble wand and wave it in the air to singing or music.

Streamers

Waving a streamer through the air develops movement and strength in the shoulders, and it is fun! You can make a streamer out of crepe paper or a strip of light material, about three to eight feet long, depending on your child's height. He should be able to lift the streamer off the floor and keep it up when waving it. If it is too long, it will drag on the floor and won't be as much fun! Secure the end of the strip to a six- to ten-inch length of dowel, or to an empty paper towel roll. Hold the dowel to wave the streamer to music, or wave it outside in the wind. Streamers are used in rhythmic gymnastics and are also commercially available.

Bubble Wands

Have your child dip a wand of any size (there are some very large bubble wands) in the bubble solution. Show him how to hold it up in the air and either wave his arm or hold his arm up steady and run around to push the air through to create the bubbles.

Turning a Skipping Rope

Even if your child cannot jump rope yet, he can turn the rope for other children. His body provides stability while the arm moves through a full circular movement at the shoulder. Turning a rope can be quickly tiring (try it yourself!), and it is a good idea to frequently change arms. Also, guide your child to change from an inward to an outward movement.

Wii and Other Similar Games

There are many Nintendo Wii games appropriate for children in which the player holds the controller (Wii remote) in one hand, and the screen reflects the movements in the controller's sensor. Making the arm movements involved in *Wii* activities requires a lot of postural stability and adjustment, as the child uses visual feedback to adjust the body position and arm movement to play the game. The complexity of the game and fine motor requirements can be adjusted as the child grows. For young children, it is best to do the games that just require a wave of the remote. Later, the child may be able to use more complex movements, such as waving the sensor, while also pressing directional arrows with the thumb.

Pouring

Whether your child is pouring in the bathtub, at a water table at school, or while watering plants at home, his body provides the stability while his arms develop the controlled movement for pouring, eventually without spilling. Here is the progression of steps in learning to pour, beginning with activities appropriate for toddlers and progressing to those appropriate for older children:

1. Play pouring games in the bathtub with fun colorful bath toys such as a small watering can.

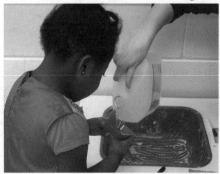

Holding a cup or bowl while liquid is poured into it helps the child learn to adjust to the changing weight she is holding.

2. Standing at a water table or sink, your preschooler can scoop and pour water back into the basin.
3. Your child holds a cup or container steady while you pour liquid into it.
4. Your child can pour water from one container into another, or into a toy such as a water wheel. Continue to do the pouring at a sink, water table, or in the bathtub, so it doesn't matter if there is spilling.
5. The beach or sandbox is another fun place to practice pouring without worrying about spilling. If a bucket of water is handy be-

side the sandbox, your child can scoop water into a smaller pail or watering can to do his pouring.

6. Let your child help you pour ingredients into the bowl when cooking or baking. Dry ingredients pour more slowly than water, and thus are easier to control. Let your child practice pouring dry things like rice, cornmeal, etc. into a cup in preparation for pouring liquids into cups.

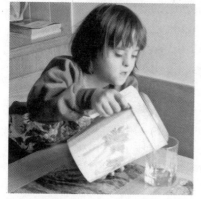

Pouring helps the child develop body and shoulder stability while learning to control movements of the arm and hand.

7. Put some liquid into a small jug with a sturdy handle when practicing pouring into a cup. Make sure your child is sitting or standing in a sturdy position. The table height should be at elbow level or lower to give him room to lift his arms up to pour. The jug from a child's tea party set may be the right size, although the cups will probably be too small!

8. Eventually your child will be ready to attempt pouring from a regular-sized jug or container into a glass.

Ball Skills

When bouncing, throwing, and catching a ball, your child uses the stability in his body as a base upon which to move his arms and hands. Ball skills are challenging because they involve a moving object, the ball. Learning to catch a ball can be very challenging for young children with Down syndrome. They must learn to plan their arm and hand movements so their hands are at the right place at the right time to catch the ball. The following progression is recommended to build success, beginning

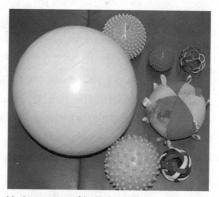

Various types of balls for ball play, including "Oball," cloth ball, sensory knobby balls, and gym exercise ball.

with activities for toddlers and preschoolers, and progressing to activities for the older child:

1. With your toddler, roll a large ball back and forth while sitting on the floor. A soft ball that will not hurt him should he miss it is best. Try a Nerf ball, "Gertie" ball, "Oball," or soft plastic ball. Some balls have squeeze-activated LED lights to help young children with visually tracking the ball. Other balls make sounds, such as the "giggle ball."

2. Many children find it easier to begin with balloons rather than balls when learning to catch and throw. Balloons move more slowly and allow much more time for the child to coordinate his movements. Try to find sturdy balloons that do not break easily, 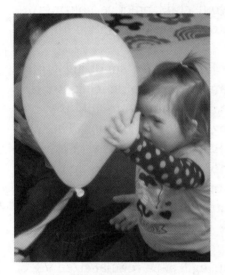 or use a fabric balloon cover that protects the balloon. Begin gently tossing the balloon back and forth in either sitting or standing, depending on your child's balance. You can also experiment with the best size for your child by blowing the balloon up to various sizes. Be careful not to leave your child alone with the balloon, if there is a possibility he might put it in his mouth.

   When your child can catch balloons easily, progress to a soft, mid-sized ball that does not have a slippery surface. Gertie balls, Oballs, sensory balls, and knobby balls are all good choices, as their grooved surfaces make it easier for the child to grasp. Stand a few feet away and gently toss it back and forth. Your child will not have good aim initially, so be prepared to chase down a few balls!

3. Some children find it easier to catch a beanbag than a ball. It has a different shape and more weight, and some children may be more successful with it. To make a beanbag, sew together three sides of two squares of durable fabric, fill with dried beans or peas, then sew up the fourth side.

4. When your child is able to catch and toss a ball or beanbag two or three feet with some consistency, stand further apart. Bounce the ball on the ground to your child. This gives him more time to prepare for the catch. Use large rubber balls that are typically used in school gym classes.

5. When your child can catch a bounced ball with some consistency, try tossing it from the same distance. Tennis balls used in children's tennis programs, which are larger than usual tennis balls and made of high density foam, are good balls to use to learn to catch when bounced. Your child should now be ready to bounce the ball at his own feet and catch it. Again, his aim may not be good at first, and he may bounce the ball on an angle, so that it bounces away from him. If this is the case, show him how to drop the ball, without trying to catch it, until he can bounce it straight down.

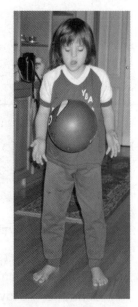

6. Progress to smaller balls, such as a regular tennis ball.
7. Your child may enjoy a variety of ball activities, such as basketball (a child-sized set will work best), or Velcro ball set.
8. As your child and adolescent gains skill, he may enjoy sports like basketball, baseball, bowling, and bocci ball, all of which build skills on the foundation of stability.

In all these activities listed above, the child is developing balance while learning to move his arms and hands with more accuracy and control. In order for him to freely move the arms and hands through space with precision, his body has to provide a stable base. While his arms are moving, the muscles of his back, tummy, chest, and neck are holding and adjusting to the slight changes of body position.

2. Shoulder Stability

The muscles of the abdomen, back, and shoulders provide the base for the child to perform accurate movements with his arms and hands. A pianist positions and holds his arms from the shoulders and elbows, while performing intricate movements with his fingers and wrists. This is the same kind of stability needed by the young child building a tower of blocks, who needs to position from the shoulder, elbow, and wrist while accurately placing one block on top of the other with his hands. Also, shoulder stability helps to keep the arms steady while the body is moving. When you carry a bowl of soup to the table, stability in your shoulders, arms, and wrists helps you to hold the bowl steady while you walk. Doing activities to help your child develop shoulder stability lays the foundation for fine grasping skills.

Lifting and Stacking

Controlled positioning of the shoulders is required in order to pick up and accurately place objects at various heights. Some activities that involve these movements include the following:

1. Picking up large blocks, such as those pictured here, and stacking them in a tower or structure or placing them down on the floor in a row
2. Placing large stuffed animals on the floor, up on a bed, etc.

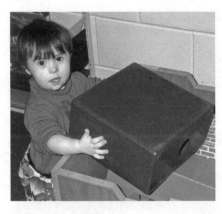

Picking up and stacking large blocks helps develop body and shoulder stability and is a good bilateral activity. Shoeboxes can be used instead of blocks.

3. Reaching up to get something off a high shelf
4. Stacking piles of newspapers, cardboard boxes, etc.
5. Putting away groceries of various sizes and weights
6. Stacking small objects such as blocks

Hammering/Banging Activities

Trying to hit a target with a toy hammer or mallet helps children develop accuracy in their arm movements, while stabilizing with their body and shoulder. Examples of toys for practicing this skill include the Tap 'n Turn Bench (with pegs and plastic mallet), Activity Hit a Ball (tapping a ball with the mallet causes it to roll down a ramp), and toy workbench or carpentry sets. Games such as Don't Break the Ice promote stability and control of shoulder movement by directed hammering.

Similarly, banging a drum with the hands or with the drumstick requires stability of the body and shoulder while the arm and hand moves to the target (the drum).

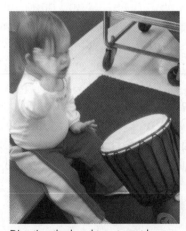

Directing the hand to a target by banging a drum.

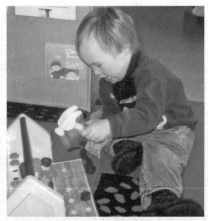

Hammering develops motor accuracy as the child targets the pegs with the mallet.

Climbing

When climbing on a jungle gym or on furniture, your child uses his arms to help pull his body up to a higher level.

1. Climbing on furniture: You can encourage this by removing sofa cushions to make the height of the sofa more accessible to your

child. Your child can be encouraged to climb on furniture even before he can walk. You must supervise him closely at this stage, as young children need help to discriminate what is safe to climb up on and what isn't! Appropriate climbing experiences include climbing up onto sofa cushions placed on the floor; climbing onto the sofa; climbing into small child-sized chairs; climbing onto a low bed; and climbing on a soft play playground. Regular height furniture will challenge your child to use more arm strength and shoulder stability to climb up.

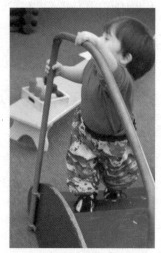

2. Climbing stairs: When your child knows how to climb onto cushions and low furniture, he can begin to learn to crawl up stairs. He will have to do this with close supervision to ensure safety.
3. Playground equipment with platforms: When your child is safe climbing onto furniture at home, he can begin to try to climb up onto platforms at playgrounds.

Using arms to help climb stairs develops shoulder stability.

Arm Weight Bearing

Activities in which children hold up some or all of their body weight with their arms require good shoulder stability. Here are examples for the older child:

1. Push-ups
2. Wheelbarrow walks (walking on hands with someone holding the feet up); begin by supporting all of your child's lower body weight by holding his upper thighs; progress to holding his feet.
3. Playing Twister
4. Yoga postures

Swinging from a Bar

Your child can begin by swinging from railings, as these are usually lower to the ground and thus safer. As his strength and overall coordination improves, he may be able to swing from a monkey bar at a higher height, and later to move from one bar to another across a row of bars. You can help your child by hugging his hips and legs as he holds the bars and moves across, so that you are supporting most of his body weight. Gradually reduce the amount of support you give as he develops better strength in his arms to hold himself. You can also use a securely fastened trapeze bar positioned at a height that allows your child to hold on and swing his legs, while still being able to touch the ground.

Caution: If your child has very low muscle tone, activities involving swinging from a bar may not be advised, as his shoulder muscles may get over-stretched. Please consult a physical or occupational therapist if in doubt.

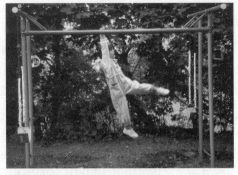

Swinging along a set of monkey bars is a very challenging activity for children with Down syndrome, as it requires a lot of shoulder stability, strength, overall coordination, and confidence.

Carrying Activities

When carrying a tray or plate of food, children need to hold their arms steady to keep the tray level and steady while walking.

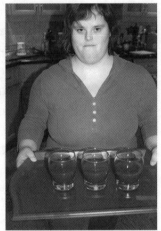

1. Begin with the tray or plate alone, without anything on it. Next, place something small on the tray while your child carries it.
2. Next, your child can carry plastic plates, cups, or other similar objects on a tray.
3. Next, your child will be able to carry a tray with non-liquid food on it.
4. Next, she will be ready to attempt carrying a tray with liquid, and later may be able to carry a tray with food and drink up a flight of stairs.

Profile: David

(Throughout the book, examples of how some of the suggested activities can be incorporated into daily routines will be given through brief profiles of children.)

Eight-year-old David goes to the grocery store with his mother. When they park, she gives him the coins to put in the parking meter. (This lets David practice dexterity.) In the store, David pushes the cart around the aisles if it isn't too busy. (He is developing stability in his shoulders and strength in his arms as he pushes and maneuvers around corners.) His mother lets him lift some of the boxed items off the store shelves and put them in the cart. When they get home, David carries some of the lighter bags into the house, and helps to unload and put away the groceries. (Lifting and carrying also develop stability and strength.)

Grandma's and Grandpa's List

- Inflatable roll: for baby to roll over, pushing off with arms and legs
- Walking toys, sometimes called activity walkers
- Push/pull and ride toys, e.g., toy doll stroller; grocery cart; lawn mower
- Hammering toys and games
- Toy trucks and action wheels
- Spinning top (spins when button on top is pushed down)
- Wagon for pushing and pulling (also handy for longer walks with children who tire but are too big for a stroller)
- Pails and shovels of various sizes
- Child-sized broom, rake, snow shovel
- Water and bath play toys for pouring
- Child's tea set with tray
- Trapeze bar
- Balloons; fabric balloon cover
- Beanbags
- Easy-to-grasp ball (e.g., Ball Jellies; Gertie ball; Oball; knobby ball)
- An assortment of regular balls of various sizes
- Child's basketball set; hockey net, stick and ball; and other ball activities
- Large blocks (shoeboxes are an alternative)
- Skipping rope
- Streamers
- Twister game
- Butterfly net
- Bubble wands

6

The Second Building Block:
Bilateral Coordination

Bilateral coordination refers to the coordinated use of both sides of the body. The ability to use the two hands together in a coordinated manner leads to efficiency and competency in fine motor skill development. Young children naturally explore and play with toys using both hands. This allows them to develop variety in how they manipulate and explore the toys. The way your child uses her hands together during play is important because it leads to the natural development of handedness (being right or left handed). This is also called "dominance." Most people use one hand as the dominant hand and have better skill and more speed with that hand compared to the other hand.

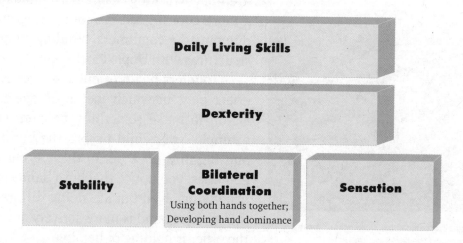

Daily Living Skills

Dexterity

Stability

Bilateral Coordination
Using both hands together;
Developing hand dominance

Sensation

How Children Develop Bilateral Coordination

An infant begins to move objects back and forth from hand to hand in the first year. This is called *transferring*. Practicing transferring helps babies to develop these important skills:

- grasping and releasing patterns as the object is passed from one hand to the other;
- eye tracking as the eyes follow the path of the object;
- bringing the hands together in midline;
- coordinating the two sides of the body.

During a baby's first year, you often see her passing toys back and forth from hand to hand as the baby carefully looks at the toy during play. At this stage she likes to shake, bang, and throw the toys. Coordination of the two sides of the body is also very evident when the child develops crawling, alternating arm and leg movements on hands and knees to move herself forward. Some children who have Down syndrome do not crawl; they scoot on their bottoms. Crawling is important for bilateral coordination, shoulder stability, and arm and hand strength.

This is how bilateral coordination develops in fine motor skills:

- Both hands do the same or similar actions (symmetrical).
- One hand stabilizes or holds the object; the other hand manipulates.
- Both hands move and manipulate, doing different things (asymmetrical).

In early bilateral coordination activities, both hands are being used to do the same thing, such as banging on pots and pans. In the toddler years, children play with toys using both hands in a more coordinated fashion: lifting and dumping out containers, building simple structures with Duplo blocks, etc.

Toddlers begin to engage in cause-effect play, in which they do a specific action to make something happen. For example, your child pushes the button, and Big Bird pops up. In these types of activities, you notice that both hands are usually involved but are doing different things. One hand is more actively doing; the other is holding or helping.

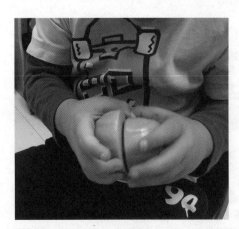

Symmetrical bilateral coordination (both hands performing the same action.

The most difficult bilateral activities are those in which each hand does a different action. Cutting out shapes with scissors is an example of this type of bilateral coordination. While one hand holds and manipulates the scissors, the other hand holds and turns the paper to allow the shapes to be cut out accurately. Many self-care activities, such as getting dressed, involve the coordination of different movements in each hand.

It can take several years for children to develop a clear preference for one hand. Even when a preschooler seems to be right handed, it is quite common to see her switching to the left hand, particularly in new activities. During these preschool years of explorative play, the child gradually develops one hand as a consistent "doer" and the other as a consistent "helper." In other words, she develops handedness, or a dominant hand.

How Children with DS Develop Bilateral Coordination

Sometimes young children with Down syndrome have difficulty coordinating both hands together during play. This may be due to poor body stability or developmental immaturity.

Poor Body Stability

Poor body stability is probably the most common reason that children with Down syndrome have difficulty with bilateral coordination. If your child needs to use one hand for balance, due to low muscle tone and poor body stability, she will have only one hand free for play. In this situation, your child cannot use both hands to hold and manipulate a toy in midline, which is a very important step in the development of bilateral hand skills.

Even if your child doesn't need to put one hand down for balance, poor body and shoulder stability may prevent her from reaching out. She may lock her upper arms at her sides in an attempt to stabilize, so that she has a very limited range for hand play. Poor balance and stability may also prevent a child from crossing the midline (center) of her body when reaching. This may affect the child's ability to develop hand dominance (34).

Developmental Immaturity

Delays in development may affect the development of your child's ability to coordinate movements of both his hands and to establish hand dominance. There is great variation in the age of development of hand dominance in children with Down syndrome, with anywhere from twenty-four months to six or seven years being possible.

It is normal for children to switch hands during activities in the preschool years, especially when they are learning a new skill, such as coloring or cutting. These activities are very challenging at first, and it is both normal and appropriate for your child to experiment by switching hands, even if you think that she is really "right handed" or "left handed."

There is no detriment to being left handed, other than needing some left-handed utensils, such as scissors and can openers. There is a slightly increased incidence of left handedness in children with Down syndrome (81).

Delays in Hand Dominance

In my experience, children with Down syndrome tend to develop a hand dominance concurrent with the rest of their development. There are a number of possible reasons why some children are delayed *beyond the normal range in the acquisition of hand dominance,* or do not seem to develop dominance at all. Observation of your child during play and activity may help you rule out some possible factors:

1. **Body Stability:** Does your child attempt to use only one hand (when it is a two-handed activity) because she is using her other hand for balance? Or, is she limited in her reach because of balance concerns, and can't reach across her body to pick something up? If so, try a more stable position for the activity, and see if that helps her to use both hands more freely.

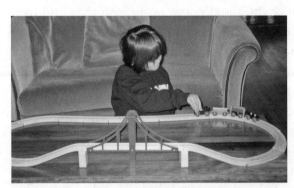

While pushing the train around the track, this child crosses the midline with her hand. This type of activity can help children who have trouble establishing hand dominance and who avoid crossing the midline.

2. **Difficulty Crossing the Midline:** Some children have difficulty crossing the midline of their body and thus will switch the toy or object from one hand to the other when they get to a point at the midline of their body. For example, a child who has difficulty crossing the midline may pick up a pencil if it is on her left side and will begin to print with the left hand, but will switch to her right hand when she gets to the middle of the paper. This is really only a notable observation if your child does this in all activities when they are familiar to her.

3. **Ambidextrous:** Some people are ambidextrous, using one hand for some activities, and the other for different tasks. Development of consistent hand dominance is only a concern if the child is hav-

ing difficulty developing enough skill with either hand to be able to function in her everyday life.

4. **Vision:** A visual problem such as a "lazy eye," myopia (near-sightedness), or strabismus may affect the development of eye-hand coordination. It is probably unrelated to the development of hand dominance.

Helping Your Child Develop Bilateral Coordination

Positioning

When your child is an infant, make sure she is positioned so she can bring both hands together in the midline, where she can see them (see Chapter 4). It is crucial that your child have the opportunity to play in a supported sitting position from a young age. A child with Down syndrome may not have the balance to sit unsupported on the floor until she is twelve to eighteen months old. This should never prevent her from sitting and developing important bilateral hand skills through play. Make good use of your infant seat and highchair!

Reaching, Transferring, and Holding

At approximately six to twelve months of age, your child should begin to pass toys from one hand to the other (*transferring*). Help her do this if she doesn't do it on her own, by bringing the toy in her hand to the center in front of her, and guiding her other hand to grasp and take the toy. The release from one hand to the other should take place in the midline, with your baby watching her hands.

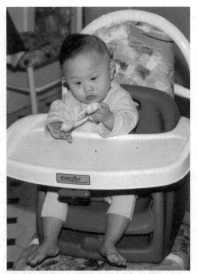

Transferring the toy from one hand to the other.

Holding a Bottle/Cup

Babies usually start to hold their own bottle in their first year. Help your baby do this, holding hand over hand. You may find that your baby doesn't have the strength to hold the bottle up herself (I found this with Sarah for the longest time), but placing your child's hands on the bottle helps her develop bilateral coordination. Eventually, although I didn't think it would ever happen with Sarah, your baby will be able to hold her bottle!

A plastic bottle is lighter than glass. It may help to use a small (four-ounce) bottle or the kind with the space in the middle, with two easily grasped sides. There are also angled bottles (e.g., Playtex angled bottle), which the baby can hold closer to her chest, rather than holding it up straight, which takes more strength. For the older baby, there are now nonspill bottles with straws rather than nipples, which also don't have to be held straight up.

Stability Activities

Some of the activities described in Chapter 5 on stability are also good for practice with both hands working together, doing the same action. For example, you can work with your child on lifting and placing large blocks or boxes or catching a balloon or large ball.

Apart/Together Activities
Clapping Games

Clapping games such as pat-a-cake are early bilateral coordination activities that bring the hands together in midline. There are many songs that encourage clapping (such as "If You're Happy and You Know It, Clap Your Hands"), and of course, we can clap to any rhythmic music.

Banging Toys Together

By about eight to fifteen months of age, your baby will be ready to pick up two small toys at the same time. Toys that she can bang together help her develop early skills in coordinating both hands together (for example, toy musical instruments and blocks).

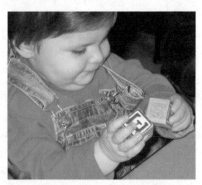

Apart/Together Toys

Simple toys that can be taken apart and

Banging two objects together is an early skill in coordinating the two hands.

put together help children begin to coordinate the movements of both hands in the midline. Some examples are:

1. Taking tops off markers.
2. Pulling apart and putting together travel toothbrush holders. These are plastic containers that hold a toothbrush; interesting objects can also be placed inside to spark your child's motivation to open one up!
3. Velcro toy food (food items that are cut in half and joined with Velcro: good for apart/together and for matching the two halves together)
4. Pop-part beads. These are large plastic beads that fit together with a little knob in a hole. They require some strength to take apart and to push together, and I have found that they can be frustrating

for children with low muscle tone until they have enough strength to manage them.

5. Magna Tiles or Magna Blocks: Colorful tiles/blocks that stick together magnetically.

6. Bristle blocks. These are blocks with plastic "bristles" all over them that easily fit together. Begin by simply pushing together and pulling apart two blocks. Later your child can attempt to put more blocks together.

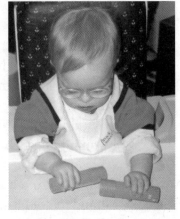

Try these activities, some of which also work on size discrimination, with your school-aged child:

- barrels
- stacking cups
- Russian dolls
- Megablocks
- Duplo; Lego
- bubble tumblers with a slot for the wand to fit inside
- train track sets

A toothbrush holder is a handy item for a child to practice holding with both hands, taking apart, and trying to fit together.

Sports and Recreation Activities

Sports activities in which both hands are used together, such as swinging a baseball bat or using a hockey stick or golf club, help develop bilateral coordination and stability.

Play-Doh activities

You can encourage your child to use a variety of coordinated hand movements to play with Play Doh. For example, she can roll it with a rolling pin, press and cut out shapes, roll it into balls, cut it with a play knife, etc.

Bilateral Activities: Hands Doing Different Actions

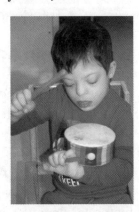

Musical Instruments

Playing musical instruments usually provides opportunities for bilateral coordination. Your child can use two hands to bang on a drum, hold a stick in each hand and strike them together, use both hands to press the keys on a keyboard, etc.

Books

Holding a book with one hand while turning pages with the other hand encourages bilateral coordination. Board books for young children are easiest for page turning. Don't worry if your child initially turns several pages at once. She will not have the finger dexterity yet to isolate individual pages, even with a board book.

As your child gets older and progresses to using regular books, she may have difficulty turning the individual pages. You can add tabs to the edge of the pages or glue a bit of sponge between the pages to separate them so they can be more easily turned.

Toys with Moving Parts

If you browse the shelves of your local toy store, you will probably find a variety of toys that require two-handed operation. Some examples include the following:

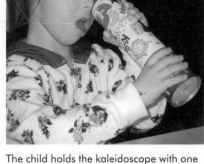

The child holds the kaleidoscope with one hand and turns with the other. The open, encircling hand position helps develop thumb positioning and control.

- Wind-up toys: Toys that are wound up, such as a jack-in-the-box or a music box, require one hand to wind it up and the other hand to hold it steady.
- Kaleidoscope: One hand holds the kaleidoscope up to the eye; the other turns the end to change the colorful display.
- See 'n Say: This popular toy has to be held firmly with one hand while the other hand pulls down the lever to start the turning dial and tape identifying animal sounds, letters of the alphabet, etc.
- Playmobil or Fisher-Price people figures; dolls
- Transformers

Self-Help Activities

Most self-help skills require the coordination of both hands. Holding the dish while eating, holding a sandwich or hot dog, and putting on socks and mittens are examples of self-help activities in which the child coordinates both hands.

Household Activities

There are many household activities that help develop components of fine motor development, including bilateral coordination. Here are some examples:

1. Sweeping and vacuuming
2. Raking

3. Folding towels and laundry
4. Opening jars
5. Using salad tongs to dish out salad
6. Using a salad spinner
7. Holding a bowl while stirring
8. Spreading jam on bread
9. Opening Velcro straps (e.g., on running shoes).

Lacing Activities

Simple lacing and stringing activities give children the opportunity to experiment with hand dominance. Usually the dominant hand does the lacing, while the other hand holds the bead. If your child switches hands back and forth when she begins doing these types of activities, it isn't anything to be concerned about; it is a normal developmental process. As she develops better control, she will probably be more consistent with which hand she uses to hold the bead and which to string with. Here is the developmental progression of lacing/stringing activities:

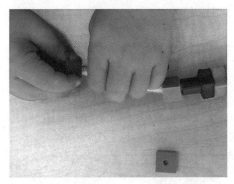

Stringing beads requires good coordination of both hands and is a common activity for developing dexterity.

1. Stringing beads with a large hole onto a straw or pipe cleaner
2. Stringing beads onto a stiff shoelace (wrap masking tape around the end to lengthen the stiff end)
3. Stringing small beads onto gimp or a shoelace
4. Lacing activities; e.g., plastic or cardboard animal shapes with holes for lacing

Movement and Fitness Activities

Yoga, dance, and martial arts activities (such as Tai Chi and Tai Kwon Do) involve moving and placing the arms and hands in different positions, and are good for bilateral coordination.

Paper and Pencil Activities

Opportunities to draw and paint give children the chance to experiment with handedness. For quite a while (sometimes a few years), a child may switch back and forth between hands with markers, brushes, and crayons. Gradually she will begin to more consistently choose one hand to hold the utensil.

Removing the perforated stickers in a sticker book requires good coordination between the two hands and good dexterity. This activity is appropriate for a child aged about seven and up, but may be frustrating for a younger child.

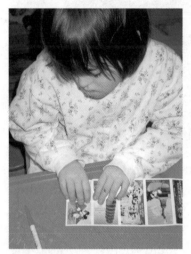

The hands each perform different movements when separating perforated paper.

Tracing stencils is another activity for the older child who likes paper and pencil activities. The child traces around the stencil with her dominant hand holding the pencil, while her other hand holds the stencil steady. You can make simple stencils by cutting shapes out of plastic margarine container lids. There are also commercially available stencil sets (e.g., Magna Doodle letter stencils) or books with stencils. Magna Doodle can be a motivating activity for the child who has difficulty exerting enough pressure with a pencil or crayon, as very little pressure is needed to make a dark line. Tracing around your child's own hand is another fun activity.

Profile: Amanda

Twenty-two-month-old Amanda is not yet walking independently, but she can push herself up to standing from her booster seat and can maintain her balance in standing while reaching. One day when her dad was unloading the dishwasher, he decided to bring Amanda over to where he was working so he could talk to her about what he was doing. He put her booster seat on the floor beside the open dishwasher and sat Amanda down in it. Amanda immediately pushed herself into standing using the sides of the booster seat and began reaching for her plastic cup. Her dad handed it to her, and she placed it down on the open dishwasher door. She reached out again, and her dad handed her another plastic cup, suggesting that she put it in the other cup.

This continued, with Amanda stacking the plastic cups, using one hand to hold the stack and the other to put the cups into each other. When there were no more cups, her dad suggested that she take them apart and make another tower, this time with the red cup on the bottom. It took her dad longer than usual to unload the dishwasher, but this spontaneous activity gave Amanda an opportunity to develop her standing balance, bilateral coordination skills, and dexterity and to hear her dad label colors.

Salad Spinner Art

Use an old salad spinner that you won't be using to wash salad anymore. Place a circle of colored paper into the spinner, then drizzle poster paint of various colors and sprinkle sparkles. Put the lid on the spinner. The child holds the spinner steady with one hand (she may need some help with this), and turns the knob with the other hand. Remove the paper to dry. The result is a beautiful kaleidoscope of color on the paper.

Grandma's and Grandpa's List

- Easy-to-grasp infant toys
- Baby bottles: small, light, easy-to-grasp shapes; angled bottles; bottle straw
- Small building block set
- Magnetic blocks/tiles
- Toy musical instruments that require two hands to play
- Travel toothbrush holder
- Play dough accessories: rolling pin, shape cutouts, plastic molding tools, etc.
- Large building blocks (shoeboxes will substitute)
- Bristle blocks
- See 'n Say
- Star-shaped rings
- Megablocks; Duplo; Lego
- Stacking cups
- Size-sorting barrels
- Size-sorting Russian dolls
- Toy baseball/T- ball set
- Wind-up toys
- Kaleidoscope; Viewmaster
- Lacing activities
- Sticker books
- Large beads; pipe cleaners for beading
- Stencils
- Sand toys
- Dolls
- Playmobil and other moveable figures
- Action figures; Transformers
- Velcro food sets (two halves of each food item are attached with Velcro; good for matching as well as taking apart and putting together)
- Train sets
- Kite with spool for winding the string
- Toy (or real) fishing rods
- Hoops; "flying" hoop
- Tool set

7

The Third Building Block:
Sensation

How Does Sensation Affect Fine Motor Skill Development?

Our hands are one of the most sensitive parts of our bodies. There are many nerve endings in our hands and fingers that send information to our brains about what we are feeling so we can move our hands accurately. There are many more nerve endings in close proximity in our hands than in our arms, legs, or feet, for example. This ability to perceive sensations helps our hands develop the coordination and variety of movements unique to humans.

The senses of touch, position, and movement, which are perceived by the sensory receptors in the skin, joints, muscles, and ligaments in our arms and

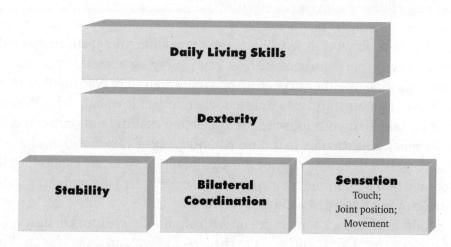

hands, all influence the development of fine motor skills. Sensation enables us to feel things, and to understand what we feel. It enables us to feel the difference between a coin and a paper clip without seeing them. It also lets us know the position of our joints and muscles even if we are not watching ourselves move. We don't constantly bump into things because our sensory systems are telling us where we are.

Sensory awareness and discrimination are important in the development of fine motor skills for these reasons:

1. They help the child learn awareness of his body for skills such as dressing and grooming.
2. They help the child learn to position and guide his finger movements so that skills such as printing, using utensils, and tying his shoes can become automatic.

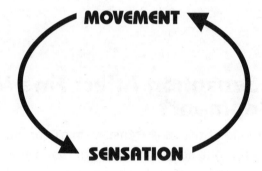

Sensory-Motor Feedback and Feed-Forward Loop

Movement and sensation form a continuous loop. Our brains receive sensory information to tell us to move, and once we begin to move, there is constant feedback from the sensors in our muscles and joints, enabling us to adjust and refine our movement accurately.

For an example of how your body adjusts and refines movements automatically, think about a time when you were walking downstairs with your vision obscured (perhaps because you were carrying something large) and had the sensation of either expecting one more step than was there or thinking that the flight of stairs was finished when in fact it wasn't. In both cases, your brain prepared your muscles for a situation that did not occur. You had to make quick adjustments based on what did occur (*feedback*), and after a second of feeling disoriented, your muscles adapted. We don't experience this sensation when we can see the stairs, because we anticipate and our muscles prepare for what we see ahead (*feed-forward*).

Similarly, if we pick something up with our hands, we immediately adjust the muscles in our hands and arms to the size and weight of the object. When we can see the object, we anticipate its size and weight and our muscles are already prepared for it before we even pick it up. If we can't see what we are picking up, we can't anticipate it, and our muscles can only react and adjust as we actually touch and lift it. If you think about times when sensory feedback from your hands was limited, as when you were wearing gloves or your hands were very cold and you were trying to do up buttons, you will know what it feels like to have decreased coordination due to limited sensory feedback. Developing good sensory discrimination is very important for our children to be able to learn to move their hands and fingers accurately.

Our brains are constantly receiving information from all of our senses about the world around us. An important part of development of the nervous system is the process of sorting out and responding adaptively to the information from our senses. This process will be covered in detail in Chapter 11, Sensory Processing.

How Do Children with Down Syndrome Develop Sensory Skills?

Young babies have better sensation in their mouths than in their hands. That is why they bring everything to their mouths. They are exploring things with their mouths because they have a need to "feel" them, but the sensory abilities in their hands aren't yet as acute as in their lips, tongue, and gums. Late in the first year of life, babies begin to spend more time looking at and feeling things with their eyes and hands, and less time exploring things in their mouths. Their nervous system is developing, giving them better sensory perception in their hands. Because the sensory perception in the hands is becoming more precise, it gives the child more information about the world.

Nervous system development is slowed down in most children with Down syndrome. Thus, hands are also slower to develop sensory discrimination. Your child may continue to put toys in his mouth for longer than usual. Sometimes a child with Down syndrome will continue to mouth things for an inappropriately long time. He can't seem to move on to using his hands for more sensory exploration. This may become more difficult to manage as the child gets older, and there are toys at day care or school that are unsafe for him to put in his mouth.

I have sometimes found it helpful to designate one or two appropriate small mouthing toys that are readily available to the child, even attaching them with a clip to his clothing (the way that a pacifier can be clipped onto a baby's clothing). The child can be taught that this particular toy is okay to put in his mouth, but other things are not. This child may need particular attention to helping him learn how to explore with his hands rather than his mouth.

When a child continues to need to put things in his mouth well past the expected age, emphasis on sensory experiences to his hands may help improve sensory awareness and discrimination, thereby decreasing the need for mouthing. Children who seem to crave chewing on toys may be seeking the deep pressure through the jaw that is achieved during chewing. Discussion of this sensory need is included in Chapter 11.

Some studies point out that children with Down syndrome may have dermatological differences (differences in the structure of the skin) that may affect how sensation is perceived. Some researchers have found that children with Down syndrome use excessive force when grasping objects, and don't adjust as readily to changes in the object's characteristics, such as a change in the weight of the object. The researchers felt this was due to a sensory deficit in the sensory-motor loop (24). In my experience, I think this use of excessive force could be due to these possibilities:

1. Children who have hypotonia have more difficulty "grading" the movements of their muscles. That is, because their joints are less stable and their muscles are floppier, it is more difficult to make the fine adjustments required for smooth, efficient hand movements

2. Processing of sensory information may be slower in children with Down syndrome. Therefore, when they are going to pick something up, their muscles may not have had time to anticipate the size and weight of the object based on the information they got by looking at it.

Children with Down syndrome will develop sensory discrimination abilities as all children do, through the experiences of their daily life. If they have opportunities to experience variety in what they feel and do with their hands, they will develop better abilities to anticipate, discriminate, and adjust their hand and arm muscles in response to sensory input.

Aversion to Sensory Play

Some children do not like many of the types of sensory activities described in this chapter. They dislike getting their hands wet or sticky. This may be due to environmental expectations (they are told not to get their hands dirty) or to a dislike of the feeling. If your child doesn't like "wet" sensory play (e.g., water, finger paint, play dough), he may tolerate "dry" sensory activities (such as sand, dried beans, or macaroni). If your child likes to put everything in his mouth, you may want to choose sensory play activities that are edible, such as finger painting with chocolate pudding, scooping and pouring with partially set Jell-O, or squeezing cornstarch and water instead of play dough.

It is normal for children to dislike new sensory experiences at first, particularly those involving cold sensations. The tactile part of the nervous system has to "figure out" every new sensory experience and determine whether it is harmful or safe. Also, be aware that the look and smell of a tactile activity can affect the way we respond to the feel of it, just as the smell and appearance of food seems to influence how good it tastes.

Sometimes, however, a child perceives *every* kind of tactile experience as threatening—even familiar experiences, such as a touch on the arm by another child. In this case, the child's nervous system may be over-responding to the touch sensation. This may be referred to as *tactile defensiveness, tactile overresponsiveness,* or sensory *hyperresponsivity.* If your child seems to feel threatened by even familiar tactile experiences, you may wish to consult with an occupational therapist, who can help assess your child's sensory and motor development and suggest a program to help. Tactile defensiveness and other sensory processing disorders are discussed in more detail in Chapter 11.

Helping Your Child Develop Sensory Awareness and Discrimination Skills in His Hands

Sensory Awareness and Discrimination Activities
Mouthing

Infants bring everything to their mouths. This is because in the beginning, the sensory receptors in the mouth are more developed than in the hands. Make sure your child has a variety of safe, clean toys to put in his mouth at this early age. Follow the suggestions in Chapter 4 to ensure that your baby is positioned to encourage hands-to-mouth activity. As your baby's hands develop better sensation, he will stop putting things in his mouth and use his hands and eyes to explore.

Appropriate toys for your baby to put in his mouth are those that are designed for infants and have the following characteristics:

- have no removable parts or parts that can break off;
- are made of a durable material that will not break down over time;
- do not contain harmful substances (such as BPA);
- will stand up to being bitten and chewed, as many children continue to put things in their mouths after they have teeth;
- offer a variety of textures (e.g., bumpy; smooth);
- are bright and colorful and offer other sensory information, such as visual and auditory (e.g., have a bell inside and different colors or shapes).

Massage

Massaging your child's hands and arms helps alert the sensory receptors and muscles. You may find that massaging your child's hands for a few minutes using firm pressure before a fine motor activity helps prepare his hands for the coordination required. Lotion may make the experience of the massage more pleasant, but it is not necessary.

Rhymes and Songs

Many rhymes and songs for young children help them learn about their bodies and hands. See Chapter 8 (page 119) for words and movements to some rhymes that infants and young children often enjoy.

Feeling Games

Games that involve feeling for an object without looking can be an enjoyable way to develop sensory awareness in the hands. When Sarah was about eighteen months old, we kept her small toys in a cloth bag. She would "choose" which toy to play with first by reaching in and taking one out without looking. For more of a challenge, the "Feely Bag Game" can be fun: Place a few familiar objects in a cloth or plastic bag, then either you or your child states which object he is going to find, and does so just by feeling. Another activity that is very motivating is opening and reaching into a bag of cookies, to take one out and enjoy!

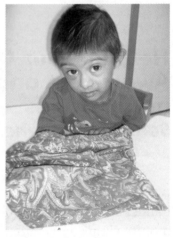

Giving the child toys in a bag rather than handing the toy to him helps him develop sensory awareness as he reaches in to pull it out.

Likewise, place little toys in the pockets of your child's clothing. Have her use sensation to reach in and pull them out.

Sensory Play

Sensory play refers to playing with any common substances and materials that stimulate many sensory receptors on a large surface of the hand. Fill a large container such as a dishpan with any of the sensory materials listed below. Be sure to try different materials from time to time for variety's sake.

1. **Dry sensory materials:** Scooping, pouring, filling, and emptying are en-

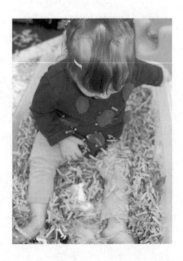

tertaining activities for busy preschoolers who get their hands on sensory materials such as the following:

- sand
- flour
- cornmeal
- dry pasta
- dry beans
- shredded paper
- wool or cotton balls
- ribbon or yarn (wrap loosely around your child's fingers and let him work at getting it off)

2. Wet sensory materials:

- water play, bubble bath, bath foam
- Finger paint, pudding or jam, cornstarch and water, shaving cream/ Cool Whip: provide a large surface (and a paint apron!) for your child to explore these textures.
- Play doh: Playing with play dough or plasticine is a sensory activity that helps to strengthen hands and fingers and encourages imaginative play and creativity. See the next page for a recipe for homemade play dough. Here are some examples of activities that develop sensory awareness and strength in the hands:

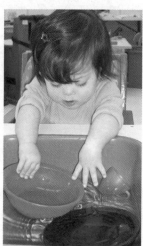

Toddlers and preschoolers love water play. Bubbles can be added for even more sensory fun.

- ❑ squeeze the play dough into a big ball
- ❑ break off little pieces and roll into small balls
- ❑ roll out with both hands into a snake
- ❑ flatten a big ball of play dough using open hands
- ❑ Use play dough tools, such as plastic mallets, shape cutters, and play dough knives; these help develop hand strength and coordination.

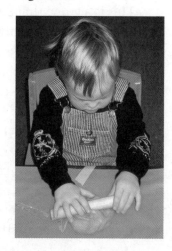

PLAY DOUGH RECIPE

Walk into any daycare and you will find play dough. It offers a child many opportunities for sensory play and developing finger movements, as well as creativity and imagination.

> 2 cups all-purpose flour
> 1 cup salt
> 2 teaspoons alum (available at drug stores)
> 1 tablespoon oil
> 2 cups of boiling water, with food coloring for color

Mix dry ingredients well. Add boiling water and oil. Mix well. Once cooled enough, knead by hand until dough is no longer sticky. Keep in a plastic bag or air-tight container.

Stickers

To help a young child learn to be aware of the different parts of his hand or body, place small stickers on his fingers, thumb, palm, cheek, forehead, etc. that he can peel off. The sticker helps him focus in on the sensation of that part of his body; you can work on body part names at the same time.

Purses/Backpacks

Many children love to have their own little purses and backpacks to carry their treasures in. These offer great opportunities for opening and closing buckles and zippers, as well as the experience of taking things in and out.

Hide the Scarf Game

This is a game that Sarah enjoyed when she was three and four years old. We took turns scrunching up a small scarf and hiding it under our clothing (inside a pant leg, inside the back of the neck, inside a sleeve, etc.). When I guessed where she had it hidden, she would have to pull it out again. It helped develop body awareness and sensory awareness in her hands.

Motion-Sensing Video Games

Several video game consoles, including Nintendo Wii and Sony PlayStation, are available with controllers that translate a player's movements into actions and movements on screen. In addition, when Xbox games are played with a Kinect motion sensor, players can control movements on screen just by moving their bodies (without holding a remote). These types of virtual reality games have been shown to help sensorimotor functions in children with Down syndrome (*85*). During these games, the child adjusts his movements to the visual and auditory feedback from the screen while playing activities such as bowling, ping pong, or golf. Be aware that any repetitive movement, done for too long, could lead to muscle fatigue and repetitive strain injury.

Using a Computer

When using a computer mouse, your child is relying on the sensory feedback from his hand position and movement to help guide the mouse while his eyes are focused on the screen. A variety of skill levels are required, depending on the type of computer, mouse, and program. (See page 175 for more details on computer use.)

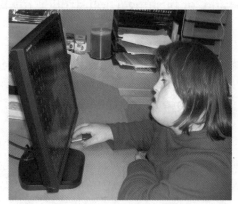

Using a computer mouse requires good sensory awareness of hand and arm position ("proprioception").

Heavy Work ("Proprioception") Activities
Pushing and Pulling Activities

Activities in which the arms are pushing and pulling (as described in Chapter 5) give extra sensory input to the proprioceptive system of the muscles and joints, helping your child be more aware of their position and prompt-

Profile: Daniel

Daniel, who is four, sits at the kitchen table every morning and watches the flurry of activity around him as his parents and older siblings hurry to get their lunches packed. Today he reaches out to help, and his eight-year-old brother hands him the bag of cookies and asks him to take out two for his lunch. He then gives Daniel a piece of foil to wrap the cookies in. His mom picks up on the fact that Daniel is interested in helping, and asks him to take out two cookies for each family member, and wrap them in pieces of foil. She then gives Daniel a sandwich to put into a sandwich bag.

Daniel is pleased to be able to contribute to this daily flurry of activity. Taking cookies out of the bag and putting the sandwich into a bag helps him develop his sensory and dexterity skills. Counting the cookies helps him reinforce counting skills and the difference between one and two. Most importantly, Daniel is learning that he can contribute to the routine and about some of the things that go into making a lunch.

ing his muscles to respond. The proprioceptive system enables us to detect the position and movement of parts of our body. Examples of activities that increase the input to the proprioceptive system include climbing, swinging from the arms, pushing open doors, pulling a wagon, carrying a pail full of sand, or pushing a doll stroller, toy lawn mower, or vacuum.

Groceries

Helping to put away groceries is another activity that children often enjoy. Picking up and carrying objects of different sizes and weights gives sensory information that helps your child learn how to adjust his movement, balance, etc., to the needs of the task. We handle a case of eggs differently from a sack of potatoes. Offering your child experiences like this will improve his ability to make the small muscular and postural adjustments needed to perform everyday tasks more effectively.

Outdoor Play/Gardening

Handling dirt, grass, leaves, seeds, etc. provides wonderful sensory experiences for the hands. Also, digging, raking, and shoveling are excellent activities for proprioceptive input into all the joints of the body and for stability and bilateral coordination. Child-sized rakes and shovels are available for younger children.

Grandma's and Grandpa's List

- Suitable toys for an infant to put in her mouth; e.g., soft teething rings, infant rattles, and squeeze toys
- Cloth tunnel for crawling through
- Stickers
- Play dough, plasticine, modeling clay, "floam"
- Play dough shape cutters, rolling pins, etc.
- Bubble bath or bath foam
- Backpack or purse
- Finger paint and finger paint paper
- Rocking horse or similar rocking toy
- Backyard swing, slide
- Sand play toys; "squeezable sand"; "sand art "
- Stuffed toys that vibrate when pressed
- Fuzzy puzzles; foam puzzles
- Touch and feel books
- Ball pool
- Play tent; adventure play zones
- Tactile mats
- Touchabubbles (thicker bubbles that float more slowly and last longer)
- Labyrinth mazes that you guide a ball through by tipping the board slightly
- Games such as Jenga, air hockey

8

Dexterity

The building blocks described in the previous chapters provide the foundation upon which your child can develop more precise hand and finger movements. We call this ability to make skillful, precise, and efficient hand movements *dexterity*.

As you can see from the activities suggested for helping to develop stability, bilateral coordination, and sensation, children continue to develop these foundations well into their school years. The smaller, more precise movements in the hands develop simultaneously, with the foundations permitting the control, precision, and speed to improve.

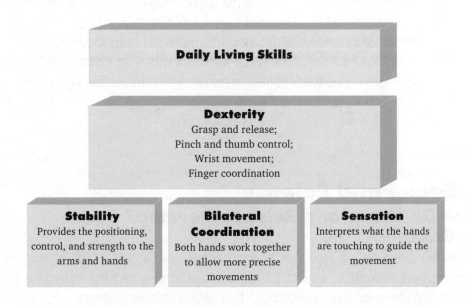

Daily Living Skills

Dexterity
Grasp and release;
Pinch and thumb control;
Wrist movement;
Finger coordination

Stability
Provides the positioning, control, and strength to the arms and hands

Bilateral Coordination
Both hands work together to allow more precise movements

Sensation
Interprets what the hands are touching to guide the movement

What Is Dexterity?

Dexterity is skill and ease in using the hands. This diagram below shows the types of movement and control that children gradually develop that contribute to dexterity.

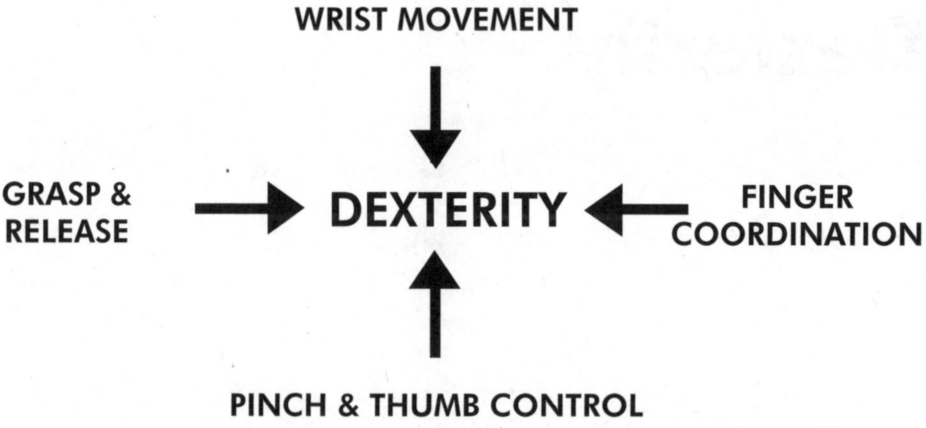

WRIST MOVEMENT

↓

GRASP & RELEASE → **DEXTERITY** ← **FINGER COORDINATION**

↑

PINCH & THUMB CONTROL

1. **Grasp and Release:** *Grasping* is reaching for, picking up, and holding an object. *Releasing* is letting it go purposefully.
2. **Pinch and Thumb Control:** *Pinch* refers to the ability to oppose the tips of the thumb and index finger in order to pick up very small objects. It is the final stage in the development of grasp and is called *pincer grasp*. To reach this stage, your child needs to develop control of thumb movement.
3. **Finger Coordination:** As fine motor development progresses, your child begins to be able to move and coordinate her fingers separately from each other.
4. **Wrist Movement:** Movements at the wrist help to position the hand for function. The wrist joint can move up and down (extend and flex); side to side; and, together with the elbow, rotate the forearm to turn the palm up or down.

Each of these areas will be discussed in turn.

1. Grasp and Release
How Do Grasp and Release Develop?
Grasp

A newborn will grasp your finger because of the *grasp reflex*. Between three and six months of age, the reflex is weakening and the baby can now grasp things because she wants to. This is called *voluntary grasp*.

For the first several months, the baby uses her whole hand to pick things up and hold them (this is called *palmar grasp*). As she begins to move the toy around, passing it back and forth between both hands (called *transferring*), and bringing it to her mouth (*mouthing*), she gets sensory information about her hands and fingers. Her first attempts to pick up small items involve using all her fingers to "rake" the item into her palm (*raking grasp*). Gradually she learns to use her thumb and first two fingers to pick up objects (*tripod grasp* or *radial-digital grasp*); next, to use her thumb and index finger to pick up objects (*inferior pincer grasp*); and finally to use the tip of her thumb and index finger to pick up even the tiniest crumb (*superior pincer grasp* or *pinch*).

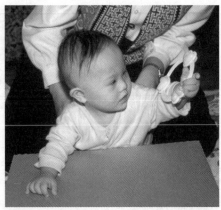
Palmar grasp.

Release

An infant initially lets go of something in her hand accidentally, without control. Usually, this is the process: your baby is holding a toy, putting it to her mouth, until her gaze focuses on something else, whereupon she immediately drops the toy. As infants, babies have to be looking at something to be able to pick it up and hold it. Gradually, babies develop the ability to pick up and hold things without always having to be looking directly at them.

Next in the development of release, the baby lets go with one hand and passes (transfers) the object to her other hand. This is the beginning of bilateral coordination (Chapter 7). Next, the infant begins dropping things purposefully; at this stage, food often ends up on

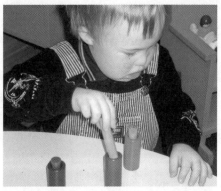
Tripod grasp of a toy: the thumb, second, and third fingers are used to grasp and release.

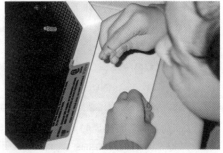
Inferior pincer grasp: the thumb approaches the index finger, but can't yet touch tip to tip.

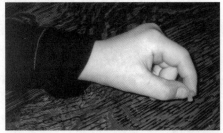
Superior pincer grasp: the thumb is rounded, allowing it to touch the tip of the index finger when grasping small things.

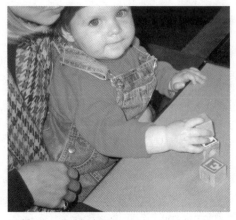
Building a two block tower.

the floor as it is dropped over the side of the highchair! Dropping and throwing continue while the baby begins to let go with more control. Now she is happy to hand you something or to release into a hole or onto a firm surface. At first, a baby needs to support the toy or her wrist on the surface as she lets go. Most babies go through this stage so quickly it is hardly noticed. Once the baby can let go of something where she wants to, she practices putting things into containers and stacking things on top of each other. By doing this, she develops more and more precision.

Progression of Grasp Development
1. Reflex grasp in the palm
2. Voluntary palmar grasp
3. Raking grasp into the palm
4. Radial palmar (oriented toward the thumb side of the palm)
5. Radial-digital or tripod (between thumb and fingers)
6. Inferior pincer
7. Mature (superior) pincer

Progression of Release Development
1. Involuntary
2. Releases by dropping
3. Transfers hand to hand
4. Releases purposefully with full-hand release
5. Isolated tripod release
6. Isolated pincer release

How Grasp and Release Develop in Children with Down Syndrome

Researchers have found that children with Down syndrome are delayed in their acquisition of grasping patterns and that there is also a difference in the quality of movements they use (24).

Grasp

Your baby with Down syndrome will probably lose her reflexive (involuntary) grasp between approximately four and ten months, when her grasp becomes voluntary. Babies with very low muscle tone may take longer to develop the strength to hold on to things. It will also be more difficult for your baby to lift and move her arms to reach for things. This is because of low muscle tone and decreased stability, as described in Chapters 4 and 5.

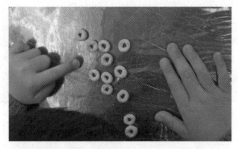

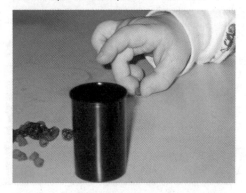

Before developing pincer grasp, the baby approaches the Cheerio with her index finger and then scoops it into her palm.

Often, young children with Down syndrome continue to pick up objects by scooping them into their palms with all their fingers (the raking grasp) for a longer time than other children do. They also use a palmar grasp to hold objects for a long time (until approximately one and a half to three and a half years) before beginning to isolate their thumb and first two fingers. They often find it hard to pick up very small objects because their thumbs can't curve to touch the tip of their index fingers. Sometimes they use their thumb and third finger together, because it is easier for them to touch tip to tip with the third finger. Usually, pinch using the index finger and thumb does eventually develop, when the thumb control and positioning has improved (sometime between one and a half and four years).

Using the thumb and third finger for pincer grasp is not unusual in young children with Down syndrome, as it is often more difficult to position the thumb to touch the tip of the index finger.

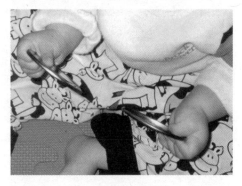

Sometimes young children with Down syndrome tuck their thumbs into their palms when grasping. This baby has one of his thumbs tucked under and the other out straight. Try to encourage your baby to grasp with her thumb out rather than tucked under.

Sometimes a young child with Down syndrome tucks her thumb into her palm when trying to pick up small things. This is a normal developmental stage that will change as she develops better control of her thumb, and can position it to touch her fingertips. If your child persists with this thumb position beyond the age of about two and a half, gently position her thumb when you are handing her something, so that she doesn't tuck it in.

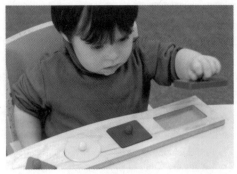

This child is beginning to orient the puzzle knob toward his thumb and index finger, but he still uses a raking motion to grasp it.

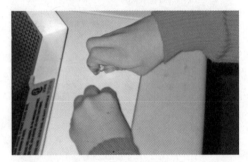

Low muscle tone and joint hypermobility in the thumb make it difficult for many children with Down syndrome to develop a superior pincer grasp with a rounded thumb.

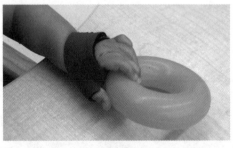

A Benik hand splint or Kinesiotape can help support the thumb joint.

Studies have found great variability in the age at which children with Down syndrome acquire the various grasping patterns. For example, the range at which a child with Down syndrome may be able to pick up a raisin with a pincer grasp is between 15 and 42 months. Don't worry if your child takes many months to progress from one grasping pattern to another, but do continue to give her opportunities to attempt the next step.

Release

Dropping and throwing are normal stages of fine motor development. For some children who have Down syndrome, this stage persists for a long time. A child's tendency to throw anything she picks up can be frustrating for parents and caregivers. Usually this is described in a behavioral context: it is a stage that the child with Down syndrome might get "stuck" in for a prolonged period of time. If a child is flinging everything, she is not able to learn some of the cognitive skills, such as taking rings on and off a peg, doing puzzles, etc., that are recommended at this stage.

This behavior pattern of throwing everything may initially develop because your child lacks the motor control to let go of things in a controlled way. She may have learned that flinging her arm causes her wrist to drop, which automatically opens her fingers and releases the toy. This can then become a behavior pattern as your child reacts to all the attention she gets when she throws things and enjoys the sheer fun of throwing. She also may not be able to discriminate between "throwable" items and "nonthrowable" items.

Some baby toys have suction cups on the bottom to keep them still on the tabletop; using these as well as large toys that are hard to throw may help reduce your child's inclination to throw everything. You can also "go with the flow": provide soft throwable toys that won't damage or hurt anyone and try to build throwing into a game, taking turns throwing or dropping, such as dropping foam blocks over the edge of the high chair into a bucket on the floor.

Your child also may need to be taught better control of releasing things (letting go), so she won't become frustrated in her fine motor attempts, such as when putting rings on a peg or blocks in a container. The throwing stage can be very discouraging for parents, but remember that it *is* a stage, and it will eventually pass. The next few pages will describe specific activities to help your child develop the skills to grasp and release.

How to Help Your Child Develop Grasp and Release

Grasp Activities
Grasping Toys

The best toys for an infant are those that are easy to grasp and pass from hand to hand and are safe to put in the baby's mouth, such as soft rattles with handles or rings. (The Skwish rattle and an Oball are two examples.) Toys are often attached to a stroller or car seat with interlocking rings, which are good for grasp development in themselves. As your child gets older, provide her with toys with a variety of shapes, sizes, and weights, so she can practice using the various grasping patterns.

Power Palmar Grasp

Your child will use a power grasp to hold on to surfaces to help her pull to stand, cruise along furniture, and climb. She will use a power grasp to encircle any cylindrical handle or toy. This will help her strengthen the joints in her thumb, in preparation for isolating her thumb and fingers to pick up smaller items. Make sure that the object fits between the thumb and index finger as it is held in the palm. As mentioned above, some children with Down syndrome tuck their thumbs up beside their index fingers as they hold objects in their palms. This can lead to delays in developing control of their thumb joints and the ability to touch the tips of their thumbs and index fingers together (superior pincer grasp).

Some examples of objects appropriate for encircling with the thumb and fingers are the following:

1. a cup without a handle, so the thumb must be placed around the cup
2. a toy plastic hammer and other toy tools
3. a plastic travel toothbrush holder

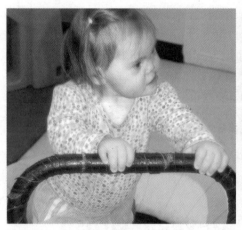
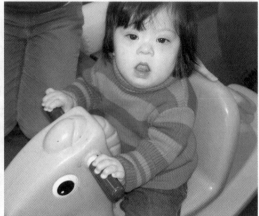

(Left) A power grasp is used to hold the bar of the trampoline. (Right) Grasping handles (power grasp) helps shape and strengthen the child's hands.

4. small balls
5. balls of play dough/plasticine;
6. any toy with a handle
7. push toys, such as a doll carriage, lawn mower, and early walking push toys.

Banging

When your baby has developed a firm voluntary grasp in the palm, she can strengthen it while learning to control her arm movements by banging a toy. She can do this while sitting in a highchair, banging on the tray, or sitting in an adult's lap, banging on the tabletop. Suitable items for banging include a spoon or rattle. Toy hammering benches (as described in Chapter 4), in which the child hammers pegs or balls with a plastic mallet through the holes, can also provide good banging practice.

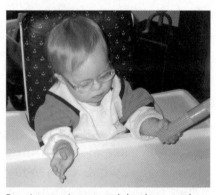

Banging toys is a normal developmental stage that helps the child strengthen his or her grasp and develop wrist movement.

Taking Items Out of Containers

Children usually take things out before they put them back in! We all know that we are more likely to find a drawer, a cupboard, or our purse emptied, with the contents scattered over the floor, than to find things around the house put back where they belong! This "emptying" stage can help your child develop grasp patterns for items of different sizes and shapes. I keep all my plastic containers in a low kitchen cupboard. As a toddler, Sarah used to love to remove them all, and carefully separate the stacks. I could see that separating one from the other was helping her thumb and finger dexterity, so I put up with the messy kitchen floor. Sometimes I would put smaller items, such as small boxes of raisins, inside the containers for her to remove.

There are countless activities at home that can give your child practice in removing things. Babies usually begin by taking parts out of containers, such as blocks out of the bin, little people out of the school bus, etc. Here are a few more ideas, progressing to activities for the preschooler:

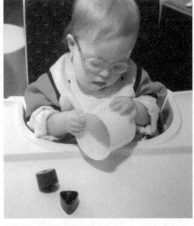

Initially, a baby will attempt to empty a container by dumping out the contents. The baby will then learn to reach in and take things out one at a time.

1. Take shapes out of a shape-sorter bin.
2. Remove blocks from the bucket.
3. Take toy people out of dollhouses, Fisher-Price bus, etc.
4. Take a peg out of a pegboard.
5. Take stacking rings off the post.
6. Take knobbed puzzle pieces out of the puzzle board.
7. Take spools of thread out of a sewing caddy.
8. Take shoes out of a cupboard and match the pairs (don't forget to try on the shoes—that's the fun part!).
9. Take things out of a "knick-knack" drawer and reorganize into categories (for the older child).

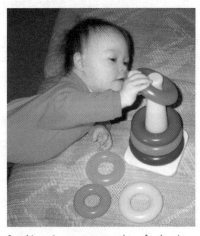

Stacking rings are a good toy for beginning to learn to put on and take off.

Toys That Promote Tripod (Radial-Digital) Grasp

Through all of the above activities, your child has been gradually refining the movements in her hands. She is beginning to isolate her thumb and first two fingers to pick up and release things. At this stage, she benefits from having opportunities to play with toys that promote this "tripod grasp." If your child seems to need help learning how to approach an object without raking it into her palm, begin by holding the object up for her to grasp. I have seen many children who rake an item into their palms when it is on the table but use a tripod grasp when the item is held up for them to grasp.

Some toy and activity suggestions to promote a tripod grasp are:

- Square blocks
- Large pegs
- Puzzles with large knobs
- Duplo and similar interconnecting building toys
- Little toy cars and trucks
- Bead tables
- Fisher-Price little people
- Putting marker lids back on (usually young children with Down syndrome use their whole hand to remove marker lids, because the lids are on too tightly for a tripod grasp to work)
- Plastic spice containers (these can be filled with something that will make an interesting noise, such as rice)
- Flat discs, such as frozen juice can lids, which encourage tripod grasp and are a good preparation for pincer grasp. You can paste fabric onto them so they have different textures. Your child can practice releasing them into a slot cut in the top of a plastic container.

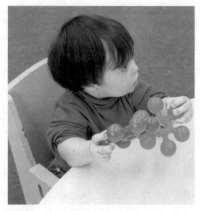

Toys such as these rings that promote opening and rounding between the thumb and index finger are appropriate for the toddler who is developing tripod grasp.

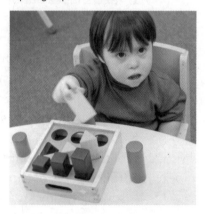

Pegs and blocks promote tripod grasp, in preparation for developing the more precise pincer grasp. Placing the blocks into the holes and onto the table helps the child refine his control of letting go.

Release Activities
Dropping

Dropping is the first stage of voluntary release. Your child opens her hand all at once to let go. She doesn't yet have the more precise movements in her hand to control accuracy. Here are some examples of activities:

1. Dropping a toy into the bathtub: This can be a motivating and fun bathtime activity. Drop a rubber duck, similar bath toy, or sponge into the water so it makes a splash and then encourage your child to do the same.
2. Dropping rubber toys onto a highchair tray or over the edge of a highchair: It can be fun for a baby to drop something over the side

of her chair and then look for where it has gone (she is also learning about object permanence).

3. Dropping a toy to make a noise, such as into a metal bowl, or a toy that squeaks when it is dropped.

"Give It to Mommy/Daddy"

This activity helps your baby learn how to put something down with control. Infants naturally go through the "give it to Mommy/Daddy" stage. They take great delight in releasing their toy into their parent's hand on request.

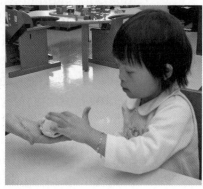

Because they need the stability, they first place the toy down into their parent's hand, and then they let go. When your child with Down syndrome is at this developmental stage, practice this skill with her, letting her see how pleased you are when she does give it to you. Immediately give it back to her and repeat the process.

Once this routine is well established, you can ask your child to "put it down for Mommy/Daddy" on the tabletop. Have your hand ready to grasp the toy as she releases

This child has just placed a toy in an adult's hand.

it onto the table. Gradually, the table will become the transition between your child and you, and she will learn that you will give it back to her by placing it back down on the table. Initially, your child may need to rest her wrist on the table edge before releasing the toy, giving her the support she needs.

Placing Items Down

Placing items down with control in an upright position is the next step. You have been preparing your child for this by asking her to hand you things into your hand. For many children, these stages of handing, dropping, releasing into containers, and placing down all seem to happen almost simultaneously, and you may

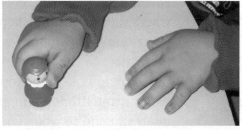

Placing objects down in an upright position helps the child develop better control.

find that you don't need to plan specific activities for each of the stages. Other children need specific guidance through the stages, as they do represent small increments in control of letting go. This may be especially true for children who have very low muscle tone and have difficulty controlling the movements of their arms due to poor stability.

I could suggest pages of possible activities for learning to control release when placing down. In general, I recommend using toys or household items that your child is interested in. Here are a few specific suggestions:

1. Place a cup down on the table after drinking. To make this more successful, pour only a small amount of liquid into the cup, and if necessary, use a weighted cup (such as a "Tommee-Tippee" cup), so that even if your child doesn't place it down flat, it rights itself.

2. After dropping toys into the bathtub, show your child how to pick them up and place them on the side of the tub. The toy is then ready for another "dive"!

3. Release a toy car at the top of an incline (such as on a toy garage set) and watch it roll down.

4. Place Fisher-Price people figures standing up on the table or floor.

5. Place salt and pepper shakers upright.

6. Set toy bowling pins down on the floor in an upright position to play a game of bowling.

Releasing into Containers or Holes

Picking up and putting things into containers is a normal developmental stage that helps children learn to release accurately. It can be built into your routine by tidying up toys when finished with them. You can also use the following activities to work on releasing objects into containers:

1. Using the same toys that your child has learned to drop, demonstrate dropping them into a box, bag, bowl, or container. For example, drop blocks into a box where they are usually kept. Dropping things into a metal bowl will make a noise that may be motivating.

2. Cut a round hole in the top of a plastic food container or a tennis ball can and drop in ping pong or small plastic balls. It makes an interesting noise when you shake it! Make the hole larger than the ball, so it is easy to get the ball in.

3. Many toys provide opportunities to practice letting go. For example, we had a Fisher-Price house with a chimney; the people figures could be dropped down the chimney and came out the other end, much to the delight of Sarah!

4. Releasing a large peg into a hole on a pegboard is another appropriate activity at this stage.

5. Shape sorters, including those that make a noise as the shape moves down, are usually too difficult when the child is just learning to let go into a hole. With shape sorters, the child has to match and orient the shapes as well, so they are good activities when the child is a little bit older and is ready to learn the concept of matching shapes. The sound shape sorters can be very motivating! Circle shapes are usually the first that children are able to match, as they are the easiest. Next are the square and triangle, and later on, the more complex shapes. Your child will probably be able to match the shape before she can orient it properly to put it in the hole. She will know that the triangle block fits the triangle hole, but may need help turning the piece until it goes in. Help her if necessary, so she won't become frustrated.

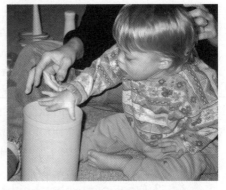

This little girl prepares to let go of the block by supporting her wrist on the rim of the container. This is a normal developmental stage in learning to let go accurately.

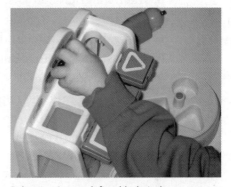

Releasing into a defined hole is the next stage in learning to release with control.

Stacking Activities

The next stage of releasing with accuracy is to be able to stack things on top of one another. How high a child is able to build a block tower is a standard item that is evaluated on many developmental tests. In typical development, a child can stack one block on top of another by about fourteen months, six blocks by two years, and ten blocks by three years.

Your child's ability to stack blocks indicates the degree of control she has achieved in shoulder, arm, wrist, and hand movements, as well as cognitive understanding of the task.

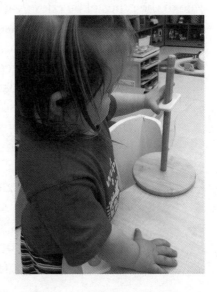

You can help your child prepare for being able to stack blocks by doing some of the following activities:

1. Stack rings on a peg. Use a toy such as the Fisher-Price Stacking Rings or a home-made alternative (see Appendix 1).
2. Stack large blocks, tissue boxes, or shoe-boxes on the floor, and be sure to give your child the pleasure of knocking down the tower!
3. Stack paperback books on top of each other.
4. Stack full rolls of toilet paper.
5. Stack magnetic blocks. The magnets hold the blocks together, so it is not as frustrating for the child.
6. Stack stacking cups, such as the Bat-tat Sort and Stack set. You may have to hand your child the cups one at a time, until she learns to discriminate size and can do them in order.
7. Stack small blocks.

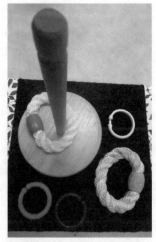

Rings of various sizes can be released onto a peg.

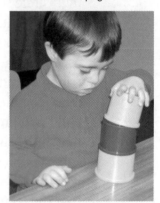

Stacking cups offer opportunities for size discrimination, accuracy of release, thumb control, and fun!

Puzzles

Puzzles challenge your child to release accurately. She also gains concepts of matching and visual perception when doing puzzles. Here is a guideline to the types of puzzles available, in a developmental sequence:

1. Wooden or foam insert puzzles of only three or four large pieces. The wooden ones have large knobs to hold onto when removing and putting the pieces back in. Teach her to remove a single piece, then place it right back in. Next, remove two pieces, and place them back in, and so on. Name the puzzle shape and describe what she is doing—e.g., "You're putting the banana *in*."
2. Foam or wooden puzzles with a few pieces that fit together to make one picture.
3. Wooden insert puzzles with more pieces and smaller knobs (such as those made by Simplex). This is often the first type of puzzle a child experiences, but it may be too difficult to begin with. Try the first two types of puzzles first, until your child gets the idea of each shape fitting in only one space and understands that she may

have to move it around a little bit so it will fit in. Then move on to the puzzles with the small knobs, which also provide the opportunity to practice pincer grasp.

4. Wooden, cardboard, or foam puzzles with interlocking pieces, in which the puzzle piece matches the picture underneath, and there is a border or frame for structure.

5. Puzzles with interlocking pieces without a frame or border. Whether they are foam, wood, or cardboard, this type of puzzle also comes in all levels of difficulty.

Profile: Emily

Emily is an active three-year-old who loves bubble baths (and since she is into everything, she seems to need one every night!). She loves to pour the bubble bath liquid into the running water in the bath, but pours too much in, so her mom replaced the bubble bath bottle lid with one from a shampoo bottle that has a flip top and a small hole. Every time she has a bath, Emily flips up the lid (developing finger strength) and squeezes a bit into the tub (hand and finger strength). She then stirs the water with her hand to make more bubbles (wrist movement, and moving the wrist and hand while keeping the shoulder and body stable). While in the tub, she enjoys "cleaning" the sides and rim with colorful sponge shapes. She can squeeze the water out of the sponges to make a rain shower (also strengthening hand muscles). Also in the bath she has squirt and squeeze bottles (hand and finger strength) and some cups and containers for pouring (wrist movement and stability).

2. Pinch (Pincer Grasp) and Thumb Control

A baby initially uses her whole hand to grasp and release things. As she develops, she begins to use her thumb, index, and middle fingers for most activities requiring accuracy and control. The most challenging grasp is the pincer grasp, the ability to pick up very small items using the thumb and index finger in opposition.

Children first learn to bring the sides or pads of their thumb and index finger together for grasp (this is referred to as an *inferior pincer grasp*). Picking up fingertip to fingertip, such as when picking a straight pin up off a table, is called the *superior pincer grasp*. This grasp is particularly difficult for children with Down syndrome due to hypermobility of the thumb joint. The thumb joint often hyperextends (bends backward) in this position, making it more difficult for the grasp to be precise. Developing correct positioning and control in the thumb joints using the previous activities for power and tripod grasps will help your child build the strength in the thumb to begin to attempt activities using a pincer grasp.

Recommended Activities

Finger Feeding

For Sarah, the most motivating activity to develop pincer grasp was picking up little pieces of food. Blueberries and Cheerios were her favorites! Other examples of food that can be used are little pieces of soft bread, little pieces of soft fruit, grains of cooked rice, etc. If your child can't pick up food from the table top, hold the piece out for her, and, if necessary, guide her thumb and index finger to take it from you.

Initially, I had to actually break Cheerios in half and soften the pieces with a little bit of milk for Sarah. She was ready to develop her fine motor skills of picking up small pieces, but didn't have the oral motor skills to manage a whole dry Cheerio. Some small foods pose a choking hazard and should not be used. These include peanuts, other nuts, whole grapes (can be cut into small pieces and pits removed), and hot dog slices. Use your judgment; if your child has difficulty with eating small pieces of food, do not use this activity.

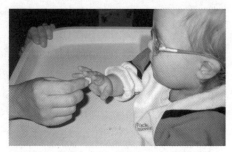

Holding up small pieces of food for your child to take from you helps when he or she attempts to use a pincer grasp.

Picking Up Small Items

Once your child is past the stage of putting inedible things in her mouth, she can play with small objects that require pincer grasp to be picked up, such as small colorful craft materials, beads, etc. This is *not* recommended until your child is at the developmental age of three years and no longer puts toys in her mouth.

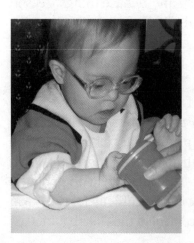

Stacking Cups

Encourage your child to separate stacking cups or plastic containers without dumping them. She need not stack them on top of each other, if this is still too difficult, but can just practice taking them in and out of each other and learning about size differences. You can make your own stacking cups with different sizes of plastic containers or plastic cups nested together.

Separating stacking cups encourages the child to use thumb and fingers in a tripod grasp.

Releasing into Slots

To release into a slot, your child must hold the object between her thumb and fingers, and hold her wrist stable. It will be easier at first for your child to put the object into a horizontal slot, rather than a vertical slot. This is because with a vertical slot, she also must turn her wrist. Adding another movement always makes the activity harder! Try these activities:

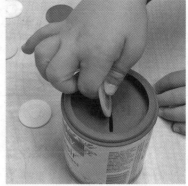

1. Putting juice can lids (or similar discs) into a slot cut into the lid of a container
2. Releasing poker chips or coins into a piggy bank
3. Putting the coins into the parking meter, pay phone, newspaper dispensing box, or other coin-operated machines in the community
4. Playing the game Connect Four

Toys with Moveable Parts

Toys that have small parts that can be manipulated or moved encourage children to use tripod and pincer grasps. Again, your child has to be able to play safely, without putting objects in her mouth, as many of these toys present a choking hazard. Here are examples of but a few types of toys:

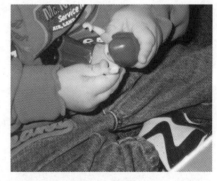

Toys such as these people figures promote individual finger movement during play.

- construction toys (such as Tinkertoys, Lego, Mechano Junior, K'nex, or Construx)
- people/animal figures that have limbs that move (such as Playmobil, Little Tykes)
- small pegboards (Lite Brite is an example, but I have found that it can be difficult to push the pegs in, which can be frustrating for the child)
- Battleship game
- Mr. Potato Head
- trucks and cars that have levers to move parts (such as a dump truck)

Strengthening Activities

When your child can use the pincer grasp to pick up and release small objects, she can continue to develop strength in this position, which will help her later with activities such as printing. Activities that can help:

- breaking off little pieces of crusty bread or bagel

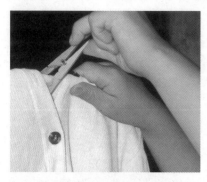

Squeezing clothespins helps strengthen pincer grasp in the older child.

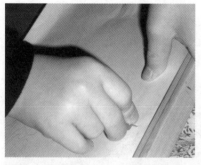

Pushing thumbtacks into a cork bulletin board strengthens pincer grasp.

- pinching off bits of play dough or plasticine
- popping plastic "bubble" packaging material (don't leave children alone with this!)
- pulling apart Lego pieces
- squeezing clothespins (helping to hang up or take down clothes on the clothesline)
- pulling caps off/on pens and markers
- poking toothpicks into a firm substance, such as pieces of cheese, marshmallows, or play dough
- games with "pop-a-dice" (plastic dome that you press on to "shake" dice), such as Frustration or Trouble
- peeling the backing off a Bandaid and putting it on a doll (or themselves!)
- grasping a zipper and zipping it up & down
- spray bottles and squirt guns: the squeezing action of thumb and fingers strengthens the small muscles of the thumb and hand. A fun activity is popping bubbles by spraying them with a spray bottle. Children can help clean windows or mirrors, or mist plants using a spray bottle.

3. Finger Coordination

One way a baby learns about her hands is by moving her fingers individually. She pokes and points and gazes attentively as she plays with her fingers. Sensory play, as described in Chapter 7, helps children develop separate movements of the fingers. Toddlers and preschoolers also enjoy songs and rhymes, many of which have actions and finger plays. I have listed some finger rhymes below. This is a wonderful stage for helping your child develop individual finger movements.

The ability to move the fingers separately from each other becomes important for many self-help skills, such as tying shoelaces and using a can opener, and for using a computer keyboard. Individual finger movement and coordination enables the child to develop "in-hand manipulation," a term used by occupational therapists to describe movements of objects within one hand, such as positioning a pencil in the fingers.

In Chapter 5, body and shoulder *stability* were discussed. When the child reaches this level in fine motor development, *dexterity,* she begins to develop the third type of stability: *hand stability*. For many daily activities requiring dexterity and finger coordination, we stabilize the little finger side of our hand while the thumb side of our hand coordinates the movement. Think of turning a key in a lock, of writing, and of using a can opener. When doing these activities, we usually keep our fourth and fifth fingers still (stable) while moving the thumb, index, and middle fingers.

Recommended Activities
Pointing and Poking

This early developmental activity is the beginning of developing finger coordination for more complicated functions. When pointing, the child begins to isolate her index finger. The index finger points while the rest of the hand is stabilized. If your child points with all her fingers extended, or uses her thumb, gently guide the rest of her hand

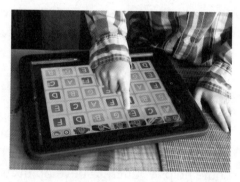

to close, leaving just the index finger to point. Point to body parts, to pictures in books, and to objects and people (e.g., "Where's Mommy?" "Where's the dog?"), and use pointing in age-appropriate iPad games, which can be very motivating. Naming objects and people your child points to encourages joint attention and language development.

When your child can isolate her index finger for pointing, she begins to poke her fingers into holes and openings. Children are quite interested in poking their finger into holes, and usually don't need much encouragement. Some safe opportunities for poking are:

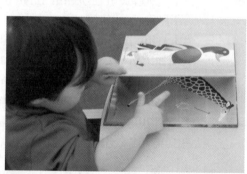

It is not uncommon for children with Down syndrome to use both the thumb and index finger to point, as seen here, or to use just the thumb. Encouraging your child to close her thumb will help her develop hand arching instead of the flattening palm so frequently seen in children with Down syndrome.

- Fisher-Price toy people, which have little holes in the bottom, perfect for little poking fingers
- holes in Duplo blocks
- preschool books with finger holes
- finger puppets
- toy dial phones
- button holes in clothing
- plastic pop bottle tops

Sensory Activities

The activities described in Chapter 7 help your child establish sensory awareness and discrimination that help her learn to recognize sensory information from the different parts of her hand. This then forms the foundation for being able to move the different parts of her hand separately, rather than as one unit.

1. When she is playing with a sensory material, such as shaving cream, encourage her to spread her fingers apart and then bring them together.
2. Weave a piece of ribbon or yarn in and out of her fingers to give her a sensory and visual awareness of her individual fingers.
3. Scoop a handful of sand or cornmeal and let it slowly run down through the fingers.

Buttons and Switches

Most children love turning things on and off. Having opportunities to do this at home helps your child develop individual finger movement and thumb-finger control. Some examples of daily home activities are:

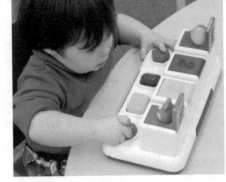

The child uses thumb and finger movement to push and turn knobs on the pop-up toy.

- turning on and off light switches (you will probably have to lift your child up to reach)
- letting her ring the doorbell when you go into your house, just for fun
- pushing the elevator button
- pushing the buttons on a phone
- pushing buttons on a TV or DVD remote, etc.
- playing with pop-up toys

Action Songs and Finger Rhymes

Preschoolers love action songs and finger rhymes! They are fun and help children imitate actions and develop finger coordination.

Begin with action songs that are familiar and are sung in preschool programs, such as "Wheels on the Bus," "If You're Happy and You Know It," "Eensy Weensy Spider," etc. Through these songs your child learns to imitate actions. When she understands imitation, and knows many of the actions on her own, you can recite finger rhymes, which use imitation to reinforce separate movement of fingers. Here are some examples of finger rhymes, in approximate developmental order:

1.

Round and round the garden
Like a teddy bear *(circling your finger around your child's upheld palm)*
One step, two steps *("walking" your fingers up child's arm)*
Tickle you under there! *(tickling under child's arm)*
(Your child can take a turn doing it for you.)

2.

I have ten little fingers
And they all belong to me *(wiggling all fingers)*
I can make them do things
Would you like to see?
I can shut them up tight *(squeezing into a fist)*
I can open them wide *(stretching them apart)*
I can put them together *(interlocking them)*
And I can make them hide *(putting them behind your back)*
I can make them jump high *(reaching up)*
I can make them jump low *(reaching down)*
I can roll them around *(rotating hands around each other)*
And fold them just so *(put them together in your lap)*.

3.

Two little blackbirds
Sitting on a wall *(lifting index fingers of both hands)*
One named Peter
The other named Paul *(wiggling each finger in turn)*
Fly away Peter *(move one hand behind your back)*
Fly away Paul *(move other hand behind your back)*
Come back Peter *(bring back first hand, finger wiggling)*
Come back Paul *(bring back other hand)*. (23)

4.

Where is Thumbkin, where is Thumbkin? *(hiding both fists behind back)*
Here I am, here I am! *(lifting both thumbs in front)*
How are you this morning?
Very well, I thank you *(wiggling one thumb, then the other)*
Run and hide, run and hide *(tuck thumbs into fists again)*
(Continue for each finger, trying to lift each individually and wiggle.
Often they are named Pointer, Middle Man or Tall Man, Ring Man, and
Baby or Pinkie.)

5.

Here is the beehive *(holding up fist)*
Where are the bees?
Hiding inside where nobody sees
Here they come, out of the hive
One, two, three, four, five! *(lifting fingers one at a time)*
Bzzzzz! *(wiggling fingers and tickling)*

6.

One, two, three, four, five *(lift fingers from fist one at a time)*
Once I caught a fish alive
Six, seven, eight, nine, ten *(lift fingers from other hand one at a time)*
Then I let it go again
Why did I let it go?
Because it bit my finger so
Which little finger did it bite?
This little finger on my right *(wiggling baby finger)*

Books

The many benefits of books for all children are well known. An early introduction to books helps develop language skills, cognitive concepts, and an understanding of the world. Books can also be useful in helping your child develop fine motor skills.

1. Board books are best for infants and toddlers, as the pages can't rip and are easier for children to hold and turn.
2. Holding a book open with both hands is a good bilateral activity.
3. Pointing to pictures develops pointing and picture recognition.
4. Preschoolers enjoy lift-the-flap books, such as the Spot the Dog books. These help children anticipate what is coming next. I have found that the flaps may be tricky for young children with Down syndrome to grasp and lift. Rather than lifting the flap for your child, either fold a corner of the flap, or add a divider tab (used to indicate sections of a school binder) to the flap to make it easier to grasp.
5. Picture books with tabs to push, pull, and turn are also readily available. It is easy to pull too hard and rip the tab. Try reinforcing the tab with Scotch tape.
6. As your child gets older, she will look at books with paper pages. When holding the book open with the left hand she gets good thumb control practice, as she lifts her thumb to "catch" the next page being turned.

Card Games

Picking up and holding cards can help develop hand stability and finger coordination. Some activities to do with cards are:

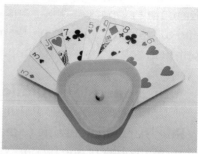

1. Pick up and put away cards one by one into the box.
2. Pick up cards one at a time and add them to the cards being held in the other hand.

A card holder may make things easier for the child who has difficulty holding, releasing, and adding cards during a game.

3. Deal cards: Even though your child is slow at dealing (goodness knows Sarah is!), try to be patient! Dealing cards not only is a good fine motor activity for the school-aged child, but it is good for sequencing and counting.
4. Fan the cards to hold while playing a game. If this is too difficult, use a plastic card holder (often used by seniors), which you can probably find online or at a toy or assistive devices store.

Games

Many commercially available games require players to use finger movements, particularly of the index finger, to play the game. Some examples are: Don't Wake Daddy; Ants in the Pants; Rebound; Kerplunk; Hungry Hungry Hippos; and games that have spinners.

Household Activities

In addition to providing opportunities for the development of stability and bilateral coordination, everyday activities around the home encourage dexterity and individual finger movement and control. When Sarah was about eight, she was keen to try unlocking the door with the key and opening the door latch, both of which helped her dexterity. When we weren't too rushed, she buttered her own bread or toast. Spreading butter helped develop hand stability, which helped her later when she learned to tie shoelaces and use a can opener. A small-sized knife with a blunt end should be used by a child.

Pushing buttons on a microwave helps finger coordination as well as developing food preparation skills, number recognition, and a sense of time. Likewise, using a TV remote control and entering the numbers on a phone help with finger control and teach number skills. Video games (used in moderation) can help your child develop better control and speed of finger movements.

Dressing

You can make a dress-up game out of having your child try on adult-sized gloves. This helps her move each finger separately into the finger openings.

Fastening zippers and buttons requires the ability to move fingers separately and to stabilize the rest of the hand. Specific strategies for dressing and other self-help activities are in Chapter 10.

In-Hand Manipulation

Collecting in the Palm ("Squirreling"). It is challenging to pick up several small objects one by one, tuck them into the palm, and hold them there. That is because you are doing two things with your hand at once. Moving small objects from palm to fingertips is called "translation" by OTs. These activities are appropriate for older children who have good pincer grasp. If your child needs to help with her other hand initially, that is fine. Some activity examples are:

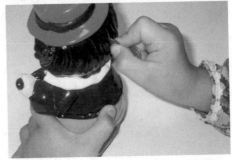

This picture demonstrates thumb rounding for pincer grasp and collecting in the hand. Releasing into a vertical slot, as shown here, is usually more difficult than releasing into a horizontal slot, because of the wrist positioning required. Once the first coin is released, the child uses hand movement to bring the coin forward to her fingertips to release it as well.

1. When tidying up small pieces of a game or toy, make a game out of it by challenging your child to see how many pieces she can pick up one at a time and hold in her hand before it "overflows."
2. Let your child help you count your change by picking up the coins one at a time and keeping them in her hand.
3. Have her pick up raisins one at a time to collect a handful for a "flavor burst!"
4. After your child can pick up and hold several small items, she can try bringing them out, one at a time, without helping with the other hand, such as we do when putting a handful of coins into a parking meter or vending machine one at a time, or when releasing marbles into a marble run.
5. Some games, such as Don't Spill the Beans, involve holding small pieces in the palm while placing them down one by one.

Rotating and Shifting in the Hand. In-hand manipulation also includes rotation (moving an object around in the hand with the fingers), and shifting (moving an object, such as a pencil, up and down in the hand with the fingers). Some activities are:

1. Adjusting chopsticks between the fingers
2. Picking up and adjusting a pencil using the fingers
3. Using "flip crayons," which have a different color on each end. Your child can try to flip the crayon around to the other end without using the other hand to help.

Profile: Alexander

Nine-year-old Alexander is the official "toast maker" in his family. Each morning he is responsible for making toast. First he undoes the twist tie on the bread bag (developing finger coordination). Then he puts the bread into the toaster, pushing down the lever (developing finger strength). When the toast pops up, he butters it using soft butter or margarine (hand stability). If somebody wants honey on their toast, he dips the knife into the honey jar and turns the knife in his fingers until the honey stops dripping (individual finger movement). Although this was a little bit messy at first, with daily practice Alexander has developed a lot more finger control, which seems to be carrying over into some school tasks, such as cutting and gluing.

4. Wrist Movement

Our wrist positions and stabilizes our hand for function and precision. Whereas our elbow only moves in and out, our wrist moves from side to side, up and down, and helps to turn the palm up and down. If you turn your own hand palm up and pretend you are catching some sand being poured into it, you will notice that your hand arches in several directions, enabling your hand to form a little "cup."

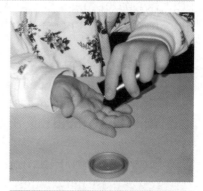

Sometimes rotating the forearm to turn the palm up and "cup" the hand is difficult for young children with Down syndrome. Often the hand appears flattened, without the development of the "arches" in the hand. This is not unusual when there is low muscle tone in the hands.

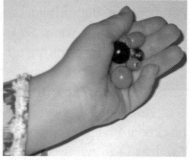

When we hold a pen and write, we usually bend our wrist up (in extension) to position our hand most efficiently. Positioning our

Placing the back of the hand down on the table can help your child hold something in her palm.

wrist in this way is a developmental progression and will not be seen in the very young child, who keeps her wrist straight. Some children with Down syndrome may not automatically progress to using an extended wrist position for fine motor activities. Because our hands work more efficiently in this position, your child's speed and control will be more likely to improve if you help her learn to position her hand in wrist extension.

Recommended Activities

Play and Eating

Toddlers start to develop wrist movement during play and eating. Your child will turn her wrist and forearm while holding something in order to see it better or to bring it to her mouth. Eating with a spoon requires wrist movement. If this is difficult for the young child, an angled spoon can be used until wrist movement develops. As she grows, she will rotate her wrist to help position toys and parts, especially toys that have interlocking pieces.

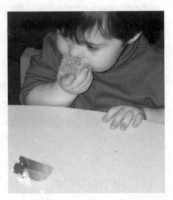

Wrist rotation usually occurs spontaneously during play and eating.

"Give Me Five"

This familiar, fun greeting encourages your child to rotate her wrist to offer her palm to get "five." You can also help her improve accuracy of arm movements by doing the "up high, down low, to the side" version.

Sensory Play

Pouring sand, dry beans, or macaroni into your child's palm encourages her to rotate her wrist and "cup" her palm. This will be easier if she cups both hands and holds them together.

Play Dough/Plasticine

You can use play dough in a variety of ways to work on wrist movements. For example, flattening a ball of play dough with the palms of the hands promotes wrist extension. So too does rolling out play dough with a rolling pin.

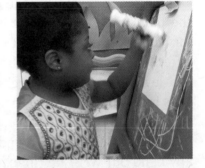

Drawing/Painting at an Easel

Using an upright surface such as an easel or blackboard helps promote wrist extension when painting or drawing. Ideally, the surface should be at your child's eye level. She could also practice the same wrist motion by helping to paint walls (you may or may not want to attempt this!).

Functional wrist position is encouraged at an easel.

Self-Help Activities

You can request the cupped hand position, palm up, from your child in many daily activities:

1. If your child takes daily vitamins, pour the vitamin (or have her pour her own) into her palm.

2. When washing her hair, squeeze the shampoo into her palm.
3. Squeeze liquid soap or lotion into her palms.
4. If she is helping you in the kitchen, she can pour the salt into her palm to put into the pot.
5. What better motivation than another child who wants to share her Smarties or M & Ms!

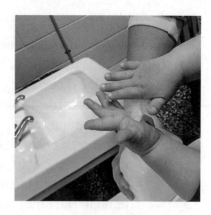

Some younger children may not be able to hold things in their palm. For a routine activity, such as taking vitamins, have your child hold the bottle cap in her palm, as it places her hand in the correct position, and enables her to "catch" the vitamin. Reinforcing this position day after day will eventually help her develop the ability to arch her hand on her own to hold things in her palm.

Canteens

There are many colorful drinking cups with lids for children. Consider getting the type that has a straw inside a lid that must be turned to expose the straw. Your child will need to move her wrist from side to side while turning the lid.

Household Activities

Some activities that encourage wrist movement include the following:

- opening jars and lids;
- turning a key in a lock (e.g., Chicco toy with keys);
- turning doorknobs;
- turning knobs (e.g., on the dishwasher or washing machine);
- stirring (e.g., mixing a glass of chocolate milk);
- shaking (e.g., shaking a bottle of salad dressing, fruit juice, or anything else that says "shake before opening");
- sprinkling (e.g., sprinkling parmesan cheese on spaghetti);
- pouring a little bit of fish food into the hand to sprinkle into the fish bowl;
- rolling out dough or pie crust;
- moving a computer mouse;
- using a hand-held pencil sharpener;
- brushing teeth, hair, pets

Toys and Games

Examples of games that encourage wrist movement include the following:

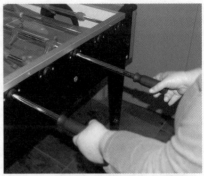

- shaking dice during a game and holding cards, which encourages wrist rotation;
- throwing a Frisbee (your child must flick her wrist down, then up);
- tossing a small beanbag from one hand to the other (to catch it, she'll turn her palm up, and to toss it, she'll turn her palm and wrist downward);

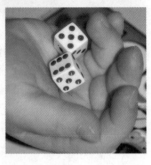

- playing with a Slinky, palms up, and holding the Slinky in both hands while it "slides" from one side to the other;
- winding and unwinding kite string from the spindle;
- playing racquet games (ping pong, badminton, tennis);
- playing Foosball;
- playing with a magnetic dart game and cocking the wrist back to release the dart.

Musical Instruments

Shakers, maracas, bells, drums, and tambourines all use wrist movement. It can be a lot of fun to join in on your favorite CD with your own instrument!

Dexterity: Summary

There are four main developmental patterns that occur as our children develop dexterity:

1. More control is gained at the wrist, leading to the ability to rotate the wrist to turn the palm up and to perform precise hand skills with the wrist positioned for function.
2. Grasp and release patterns progress from grasping in the palm to using the tips of the thumb and fingers.
3. More control is gained in the thumb, leading to the ability to position the thumb to oppose the index finger.
4. Movement control in the fingers progresses so that the fingers are able to move separately from each other, and your child can perform a variety of movements with different parts of the hand.

Grandma's and Grandpa's List

Grasp and Release
- Bath toys
- Activity center/floor gym
- Building blocks; foam building blocks
- Stacking rings/stacking cups and other stacking toys
- Shape sorters
- Workbench or tool play set
- Puzzles (large knobs; sponge puzzles; small knobs; interlocking pieces), depending on the developmental level of the child
- Toy diggers
- Baby Discovery toys (Fisher-Price)
- Fisher-Price Little People (e.g., school bus)
- Ball mazes (larger balls for younger children, marbles for older children)

Pinch and Thumb Control
- Peg boards (large pegs or small, depending on the developmental age of the child)
- Battleship; Lite Brite
- Piggy bank
- Etch-a-Sketch
- Bead stringing set
- Modeling clay, plasticine
- Stamp pad
- Duplo, Lego, Tinkertoys, Mechano, other building sets
- Bead tables (colorful beads can be moved along the interwoven colored wire)
- Tweezer games (such as tweezer marble games; Operation)
- Squirt guns; toys that shoot foam balls when squeezed

Finger Coordination
- Action figures; Transformers
- Moveable people/animal figures or dolls such as Little Tykes, Playmobil, Fisher-Price
- Dolls and doll clothes
- Simple card games

- Musical instruments (toy or real): piano, recorder, sax, guitar, or banjo
- Puppets and finger puppets
- Books: board books, flap books, pop-up and tab books, picture books, etc.
- Toy dial phone; flip phone
- Child's tape player
- Games such as Connect 4, Ants in the Pants, Ker-Plunk, Mr. Potato Head
- String art
- Gloves
- Toy cash register
- Dressing puzzles

Wrist Movement
- Frisbee
- Rainbow caterpillar (moveable gears)
- Slinky
- Beanbags
- Drink canteen
- Barrel of monkeys
- Racquet games
- Musical instruments (bells, shakers, maracas, tambourines)
- Magnetic dart game
- Toy football
- Bubble wands

Handy Basket: Toys and Activities to Keep Handy

When Sarah was young, I found it helpful to keep a number of activities handy in a plastic basket. They were ready to be pulled out whenever there was an opportunity for Sarah to play with "her basket." These pages can be copied and posted for quick reference to give parents a general idea of the types of activities that can be kept handy to help their child develop dexterity skills.

Handy Basket: Birth to 2 Years

Hand Development Goals	Item/Activity	Skills Developed
watching hands	hanging toys to reach for and grab onto	swatting; moving hands in visual field
reaching	rattles, toys with handles to grasp and shake	grasping and holding; moving whole arm; stability
grasping in palm	toys safe to put in mouth	sensory exploration
passing from hand to hand	easy to grasp with both hands	hands working together
grasping on thumb side of hand	blocks/container; large pegboard	thumb control; using fingers for grasp
placing toys down	pegs and rings	accuracy of placing and letting go
using both hands for play	simple manipulative toys (e.g., pop-apart beads, Duplo, activity boxes)	coordinating both hands to pull apart/put together
isolated finger movement	ribbon/wool/yarn; board books; toys with holes for poking	sensory awareness of fingers; pointing; poking
moving/rotating objects with hands	insert puzzles; shape sorters	finger coordination; wrist movement

Handy Basket: 2–4 Years

Hand Development Goals	Item/Activity	Skills Developed
accurate placing and letting go	blocks; stacking rings; pegs in pegboard	accurately aligning objects; positioning and releasing
using thumb and index finger for pincer grasp	picking up and letting go of small objects (e.g., raisins, Cheerios); removing insert puzzle pieces with knobs	pincer grasp and release; thumb strength
wrist rotation	pouring activities/water play; pouring objects into palm	turning forearm and wrist to position the hand
palmar grasp of crayon	preprinting activities with markers and crayons	initial developmental grasp of crayon
digital-pronate grasp of crayon	drawing, coloring, painting	next stage in progression of pencil grasp
more use of one hand as preferred (but still switches often)	activities requiring both hands, but the hands have different movements (e.g., Tinkertoys); stringing large beads on pipe cleaner	bilateral coordination; development of preferred hand
isolated finger movement to manipulate objects	play dough: rolling into snake, balls; breaking off little pieces; picture books; finger puppets; scissors	movement of small joints in hand; sensation in hand
Tripod grasp of crayon	preprinting activites	prepares hand to learn visual-motor skills such as printing; control of pencil; movement

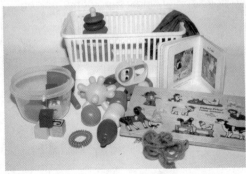

Toys for birth to two years.

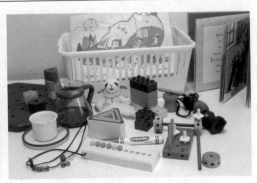

Toys for two to four years.

Handy Basket: 5–8 Years

Hand Development Goals	Item/Activity	Skills Developed
tripod grasp	Chalk, marker, crayons, paintbrushes; coloring and activity books	holding writing utensils in tripod grasp; directing strokes and coloring
wrist rotation	wallet; emptying coins to palm; small bottles and jars; turning key toy	forming "cup" palm to hold items; control of amount of wrist rotation and speed
accurate pincer grasp and release, with more speed	stringing small beads; coins into piggy bank; clothespegs; small Lego pieces	strength of thumb and index finger; faster, more automatic movements
uses a preferred hand; other hand assists	lacing activities; stringing beads; tracing stencils; sticker books; kaleidoscope; construction toys (e.g., Lego)	hand dominance; coordination of the two hands working together; assistant hand learns how to make fine adjustments
control of small joint movement	rolling small balls out of play dough; sharpening a pencil; manipulating small moveable toys (e.g., Playmobil people); fastening snaps, buttoning; zipping; drawing tiny circles; scissors: cutting corners, curves	sensory awareness of movements of small joint of the hand; strength of fingers; using different fingers for different movements; ability to turn an object around in the hand without holding it against the body

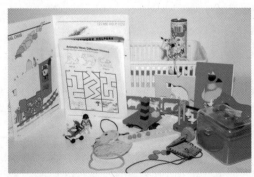

Activities for five to eight years.

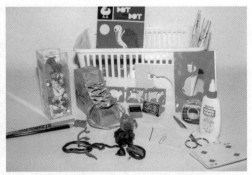

Activities for nine to twelve years.

Handy Basket: 9–12 Years

Hand Development Goals	Item/Activity	Skills Developed
automatic, quick movement of individual fingers	putting bobby pins on card; opening and closing large safety pins; tying knot in scarf or stiff shoelaces; twisting pipe cleaners together; opening and closing twist ties; breaking off pieces of tape; doubling rubber bands around a deck of cards; putting paperclips on card	precise control of small movements for functional activities
in-hand manipulation	put coins in piggy bank, taking one at a time from the palm with same hand; shuffling cards; braiding stiff laces or pipe cleaners; turning pencil around in hand to erase (without using other hand to help)	development of all the muscles in the hand
automatic visual-motor skills	dot-to-dot books; printing, drawing, or coloring; scissors: cutting small shapes; craft activities	refinement of visual-motor abilities will help develop written communication skills

9

Daily Living Skills:
School Tasks

If you look at the fine motor skills "house model," you will see that your child uses the building blocks and dexterity abilities to take on new challenges when he gets to school. School-related activities challenge children not only to use their developing dexterity, but also to coordinate this with visual and perceptual skills. The coordination of visual and motor information is called *visual-motor integration* or *eye-hand coordination*.

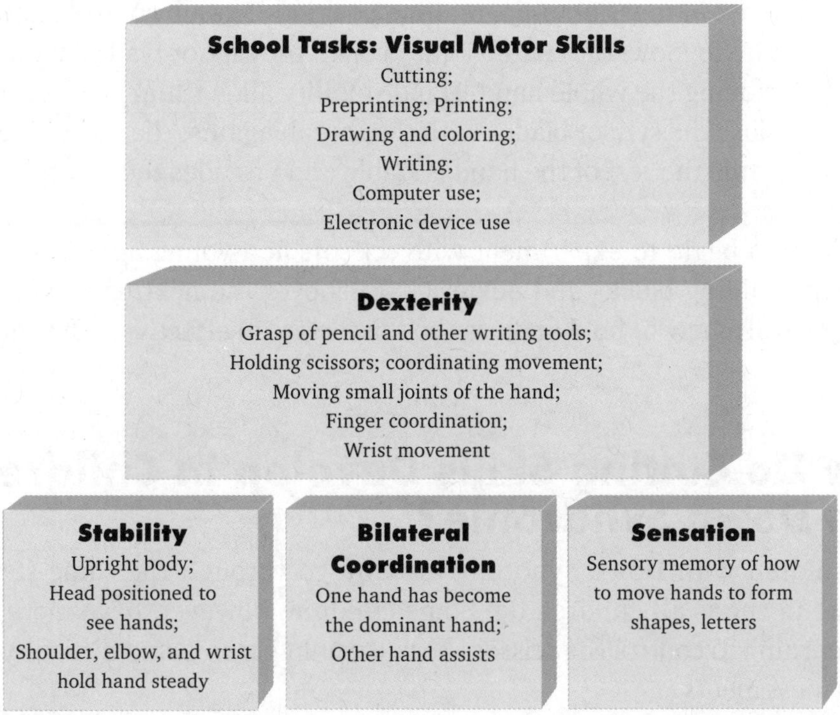

School Tasks: Visual Motor Skills
Cutting;
Preprinting; Printing;
Drawing and coloring;
Writing;
Computer use;
Electronic device use

Dexterity
Grasp of pencil and other writing tools;
Holding scissors; coordinating movement;
Moving small joints of the hand;
Finger coordination;
Wrist movement

Stability
Upright body;
Head positioned to
see hands;
Shoulder, elbow, and wrist
hold hand steady

Bilateral Coordination
One hand has become
the dominant hand;
Other hand assists

Sensation
Sensory memory of how
to move hands to form
shapes, letters

Visual motor skills are the specific tasks and activities that involve the coordination of eye movement, visual perception, and fine motor skills. Visual motor activities discussed in this chapter include cutting, preprinting, drawing, coloring, printing, handwriting, and using computers and personal electronic devices.

Let us look at how the model of fine motor skills can be applied to visual motor skills. These are the building blocks and the dexterity abilities that contribute to visual motor development.

Cutting

Cutting is a higher level fine motor skill because it relies on many lower level skills:

- **Bilateral Coordination:** The assistant hand positions and adjusts the paper so that the dominant hand can align the scissors with the paper to cut out the shape.
- **Stability:** Body and shoulder stability enable the child to make accurate movements with both hands.
- **Sensation:** Sensory feedback from the joint and muscle proprioceptors help make the small adjustments necessary to cut accurately.
- **Dexterity:** Wrist rotation helps the child position the cutting hand in the thumb-up, midline position. Thumb control allows him to move the thumb joint to open the scissor blades, without moving the whole hand. Hand stability allows him to open and close the scissor blades with the thumb against the index finger, while the rest of the hand is stable and provides the control.

Children begin to experiment with scissors at a young age. As they develop the building blocks and dexterity skills over the next few years, they gradually learn how to hold and use the scissors in an effective, efficient way.

How Do Cutting Skills Develop in Children with Down Syndrome?

Children with Down syndrome usually go through the same steps in learning to cut as all children do. Some children, however, have more difficulty learning to control the scissors because of hypotonia and difficulty with thumb movements.

When first experimenting with scissors, children often hold them in both hands. This is a normal exploratory stage. When they begin to hold the scissors in one hand, children usually use a pronated grasp—that is, with the palm of the hand and the thumb facing down and away from the body. Often the fingers are splayed open. In this position it is difficult even to snip. If your child is at this stage developmentally, do not expect him to be able to cut out corners and curves or even a straight line. It is simply too hard.

Your child will gradually learn to rotate his wrist to position his arm in the midline position, thumb up and palm facing the other hand. In this position, the thumb can move more effectively against the index finger, and more control is achieved. It will probably take your child a while to progress to holding the scissors in the midline position, and even with his hand in the proper position, he may have difficulty opening and closing the scissor blades because he hasn't yet developed control of thumb movements. A child with Down syndrome may use opening and closing movements of the whole hand until he develops more strength and control in his thumb. Some children prefer to put both their index and middle fingers together in the loop, which is fine, as it gives them more stability. At this stage, it is often beneficial to use self-opening scissors (see below).

Initially, the movement directing the scissors comes from the shoulder and elbow. Children gradually refine this movement until the larger joints are kept stable while the wrist and small joints of the hand direct the scissor movement.

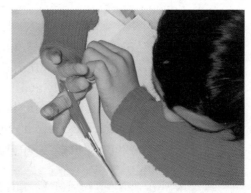

The role of the assistant hand in cutting is important, but often overlooked. Cut out a complex pattern and notice how much you turn and position the paper with your assistant hand. It is much more difficult to cut without all the adjustment and positioning of the paper by the assistant

Scissor grasp commonly seen in children with Down syndrome when learning to cut. Lacking control of thumb movement, this child uses opening and closing movements of all the fingers to operate the scissors. His arm is turned in (pronated) so that he starts cutting on the side of the paper rather than at the bottom.

hand. Holding and adjusting the paper with the other hand is difficult initially for children with Down syndrome. To prevent frustration, help your child hold the paper, or tape both ends of the paper down, leaving the rest of the paper lifted up off the table, so your child can insert the scissors easily.

Helping Your Child Develop Cutting Skills

The activities suggested in the chapters on the "building blocks" of fine motor skill development (stability, bilateral coordination, and sensation) will help prepare your child for learning to cut. In order to cut effectively, your child needs to have body and shoulder stability, and needs to be able to coordinate the movements of both of his hands. In addition, the activities suggested in Chapter 8: Dexterity, will help your child develop the movements necessary for cutting, particularly wrist rotation, thumb control, and hand stability.

Recommended Activities

Puppets

Playing with a hand puppet and moving the puppet's mouth can introduce your child to the hand movement of opening and closing the fingers and thumb that is used when he begins to learn to cut. You can use cloth puppets or puppets made from paper bags.

Squeezing Activities

Playing games that involve using tweezers and tongs to pick up objects can help develop the thumb movement and control for cutting. Some activity examples are:

1. Pick up small pieces of cut-up sponge with tongs or tweezers and then drop the pieces into a bowl of water or into the bath.
2. Some commercially available games such as "Giggle Wiggle" involve using tweezers (in this game, the child picks up and releases marbles onto a wiggly caterpillar).
3. Use tweezers to pick up finger foods, such as raisins or marshmallows.
4. Squeezing a baster or puff blower also helps develop thumb movement and strength; for example, your child can:
   - make bubbles in water with a baster
   - have ping-pong ball races, using the air from squeezing the baster or puff blower to move the ball
   - play with spray bottles and squirt guns, which use the same thumb-finger motion

Ripping Activities

Cut strips of paper that your child can rip into small pieces. Many children find this motivating in itself. After all, usually they are scolded if they rip paper! Some types of paper (such as crepe or tissue paper) have a grain, and are easier to rip in one direction. Grasping the top of the paper strip with both hands and moving the hands in opposite directions to rip it helps your child with the midline hand position and wrist movements used in cutting.

Choice of Scissors and Paper
Scissors

Choosing scissors may require some trial and error until you find a pair that works for your child. Here are some points to keep in mind when selecting scissors:

1. Your child's hand is probably quite small, so look for scissors that don't require a lot of movement to open the blades.
2. Child-sized squeeze or self-opening scissors are often a good first step to cutting for children with Down syndrome. These scissors help the child position his hand in the thumb-up (midline) position, and he needs only to squeeze them to cut. They then automatically reopen. Fiskars makes a small pair of "squeezers" and preschool scissors that

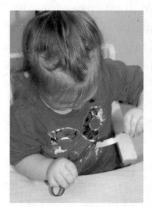
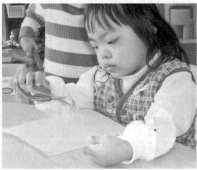

Therapro self-opening scissors are the first introduction to cutting for these children.

work well for some children. Therapro (see Resources) distributes a red loop scissor that is perfect for little hands, and is a little easier to squeeze than the Fiskars. I have found typical-looking children's scissors at dollar and other stores that can switch from self-opening to regular scissors.

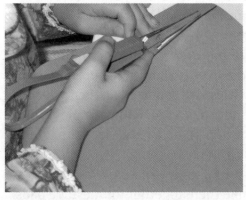
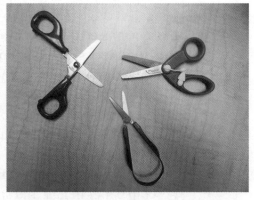

(Left) Loop (self-opening) scissors are often easier when beginning to learn cutting, as they help the child position his or her hand with the thumb pointing upward and they open automatically. (Right) Three types of self-opening scissors.

3. Scissors with double finger loops allow an adult to place his hand over the child's to assist him to cut.
4. Metal blades work better than plastic blades, but the tips should be rounded for safety when your child is young.
5. I have found that small sewing scissors sometimes work better than children's scissors, but be careful of sharp points.
6. Self-opening (loop) scissors should work if your child is right or left handed. Once he has progressed to regular scissors, you should look for left-handed scissors if he is left-handed, as right-handed scissors won't work as well and may be frustrating.

Paper

Paper with a slightly heavier weight and stiffness will be easier for your child to manage initially than regular writing paper (which is too flimsy) or poster board (which is too stiff). Construction paper is often a good choice. I like to use paper the thickness of paint samples or playing cards.

Learn Step by Step

If your child is just beginning to learn to hold scissors and the paper, don't expect him to actually be able to cut anything out yet! As when learning any skill, he needs to learn the developmental progression step by step:

1. **Snipping: short, individual snips.** Give your child small strips of paper that can be cut into smaller pieces with just a snip. This may be motivating enough in itself, or he may want to collect a pile of tiny bits, and glue them onto a predrawn picture, with a mosaic-like result. Picking up the little bits of paper is also good for pincer grasp. Another activity example is to cut a fringe with individual snips, such as to make a lion's mane, or a placemat fringe. A fringe is harder to cut than small bits, as the scissors must be placed quite accurately.
2. **Cutting across a thin strip of paper (e.g., one inch) and then wider strips.** Here your child makes two or three cuts in the same direction. He ends up with small squares of paper, which can be glued into a design or onto a picture. Paint samples (you can pick them up at hardware stores) are a good size for beginning cutters.
3. **Cutting a piece of paper in half.** Sarah and I used to cut pieces of scrap paper in half and staple them together for message pads. This was a good opportunity for Sarah to practice cutting across a piece of paper.

4. **Cutting along a straight line.** Pretend the scissors are a race car that tries to stay on the track. Staying on the track is more important than going fast!

5. **Changing direction; for example, cutting an angle or corner, as when cutting out shapes.** You can also use a "driving" analogy here. The scissors are like a car driving on the road; when you get to a corner, you stop, turn the scissors and readjust the paper, then carry on.

6. **Cutting a curved line.** Here your child has to gradually adjust the position of the scissors and paper to cut the curve. For example, cut a semicircle off the corner of a paper to make a "piece of pie." Your child can then decorate the pie or can glue several together to make a whole pie.

7. **Cutting a complete circle.** While cutting, your child has to continuously move the paper with the other hand, to keep the cutting going in a curved pattern. When children start learning how to cut curves and circles, they usually cut a couple of straight strokes, then turn the paper slightly and carry on in this manner. They end up with more of an octagon shape than a true circle. Gradually they learn how to continuously adjust the position of the scissors and paper to stay on the curved line. In preparation for cutting a complete circle, you can fold a paper in half and draw a half circle from the fold. Keeping the paper folded, your child can cut the half circle out, which will be a complete circle when opened up.

8. **Cutting combinations of corners, lines, curves, and circles with increasing complexity.** Intricate cutting patterns are difficult for many children, including children with Down syndrome. If this kind of cutting is being done in a school art class or project, precut some or most of the pattern so that your child can complete the cutting pattern with a few cutting strokes. This will allow him to contribute to the cutting aspect of the activity, without getting frustrated. You can show him how to cut off excess paper as he cuts out a shape. This will make it easier to hold and position the paper with his non-dominant hand.

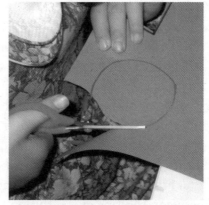

Cutting out a circle is usually more difficult than cutting out lines and corners.

Preprinting Skills

Pencil Grasp

In this book, the term *pencil grasp* is used to refer to the grasp of all writing utensils, including crayons, markers, pens, paintbrushes, etc. Children learn to hold a pencil in much the same way that they learn to pick up objects. As explained in Chapter 8, your child gradually refines his grasp and release from using his palm and all of his fingers as a unit, to eventually using very fine movements of his thumb and fingers, primarily the index finger. Your child makes the same type of progression in learning how to hold something to write.

Initially, the child holds the pencil in his palm and makes marks. This is called the *palmar grasp.* Some children hold the marking end of the pencil close to the thumb (called the *palmar pronate* grasp), while other children hold it close to the little finger (called the *palmar supinate* grasp).

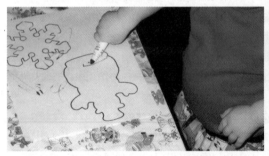 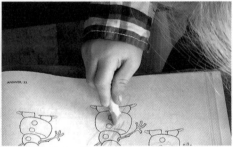

(Left) Palmar grasp is the first developmental stage in learning to use a pencil. (Right) When using a radial-palmar (or palmar-digital) grasp, the child holds the marker in the palm, but the thumb and fingers begin to position it.

Gradually, the fingers extend out on to the shaft of the pencil while it is still held in the palm. This is sometimes referred to as a *radial palmar* or *digital pronate* grasp.

Next, the pencil is brought out from the palm to between the thumb and fingers, and the thumb and fingers hold it in a somewhat clumsy-looking grasp. Most of the movement comes from the wrist and arm. This is called a *static tripod* or *immature tripod* grasp.

Finally, children begin using the mature grasp, with the pencil positioned between the tips of the thumb and first two fingers, using small movements of the hand joints to move the pencil. This is called the *dynamic tripod grasp.*

In *Clinical Perspectives in the Management of Down Syndrome,* the authors described the average age ranges for achieving these pencil grasps for children with Down syndrome as follows (76):

- Palmar Supinate .... 13–36 months
- Digital Pronate .... 24 months–5 years
- Static Tripod.........................4–8 years
- Dynamic Tripod................... 5–12 years

Although I have not done formal research to support my observations, I have found that given many of the skill development opportunities found in this book, many children I have worked with have developed static tripod grasps by the age of three years.

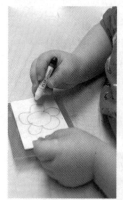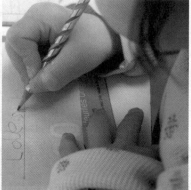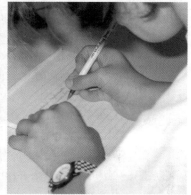

(Left) The young child holds the crayon in a static tripod grasp. (Middle) The older school-aged child gradually develops a dynamic tripod grasp, using fine opposition of the thumb and index finger to position and move the pencil. (Right) Some children prefer to hold the pencil in the position shown here, called a quadrupod grasp, as three fingers and the thumb are used to hold the pencil. This grasp works for this child.

Helping Your Child Develop Pencil Grasping Patterns

When your child is a toddler, he will naturally hold a crayon or marker in a palmar grasp. He will either turn his hand thumb-side down to color (palmar pronate), or thumb-side up (palmar supinate), or will alternate between the two. The important point at this stage is to have fun with crayon and marker activities; don't worry about how your child is holding the crayon, or what he is drawing. Showing interest and pleasure in any marks and scribbles your child makes will encourage him to continue.

Within the next year or so, your child will be ready to begin to extend his fingers on the shaft of the pencil (digital pronate). This will coincide with him using a tripod (radial-digital) grasp on objects during play, as he begins to focus on using his thumb and fingers in a more coordinated fashion. Following some of the activity suggestions in Chapter 8 (page 108) to help him develop this kind of coordination during play will likely generalize to his grasp of a crayon as well.

The next stage of pencil grasp development is switching from this digital pronate grasp, in which the pencil is positioned in the palm, to a tripod grasp. This involves changing the entire position of the pencil. It is now out of the palm and is held and controlled by the thumb and the first two fingers, and rests against the side of the hand. This is the biggest switch developmentally in the progression of pencil grasp. It is quite common and normal to see frequent switching back and forth between these two pencil grasps as your child experiments with the new feeling. Your child may begin to use a tripod grasp anywhere from about age three and a half years on. Here are some suggestions that I have found helpful when encouraging preschool or school-aged children to bring the pencil out of a palmar and into a tripod grasp:

1. Sometimes children need the sensory cue of something in the palm. "Finger crayons" can help. These consist of a round bulb, which is held in the palm, and a pointed end, which encourages a tripod grasp.

2. Use short stubs of crayons or chalk rather than long pieces. With a regular length, your child may use a palmar grasp, but when given a short piece that won't fit into his palm, he will use the thumb and fingers in a tripod grasp.

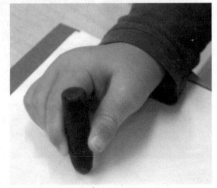

Stubby crayons promote use of a tripod grasp.

3. A triangular or similarly shaped crayon can help cue your child to hold it with a tripod grasp.

4. Thick markers, as opposed to thin, may encourage your child to use a tripod grasp.

Children with Down syndrome commonly anchor the pencil with the base of the thumb against the side of the hand, rather than using the tip of the thumb. This is sometimes known as a "thumb wrap" grasp. This is an early tripod grasping pattern seen in many children. It can persist in children with Down syndrome, probably because of difficulty holding the pencil

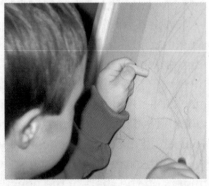

A small piece of crayon or chalk can help the child use his finger and thumb more actively.

with the tip of the thumb, due to hypotonia, lax ligaments in the thumb, and the tendency of the thumb to "collapse." This type of tripod grasp is adequate for the first few years of printing. This thumb wrap grasp may be adequate for many people, but it is usually slower than a dynamic tripod grasp. The small finger and thumb movements necessary for quick printing and legible cursive writing can be achieved with a dynamic tripod grasp.

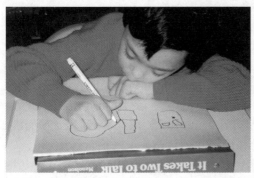 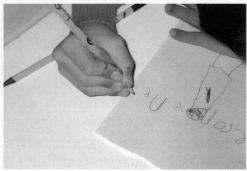

Left, a pencil grasp pattern commonly seen in children with Down syndrome, in which the pencil is anchored against the side of the hand by the thumb. Right, a pencil grip helps this child position the pencil in a quadrupod grasp.

Your child has the potential to develop a dynamic tripod grasp of a pencil if he can pick up and release small objects with a superior pincer grasp (tip-to-tip opposition). The activities described in Chapter 8 on page 127 to develop and strengthen pincer grasp and thumb control will prepare your child for making small, controlled movements of the pencil using a dynamic tripod grasp.

The progression of pencil grasp development may not come naturally to all children with Down syndrome. Your child may have to be shown how to hold the pencil the "new" way. This may mean repositioning the pencil in his hand to give him the idea. Don't be surprised if he initially rejects the new grasp in favor of the old, less developed grasp. Be aware that when he does try holding his pencil in a new grasp, he may not have as much control with the pencil at first. If he was able to draw circles with a palmar grasp, he may only be able to scribble when first shown how to hold it with his thumb and finger extended down the shaft of the pencil. However, if you consistently help him to position the pencil the "new" way, letting him readjust it after a try, he will eventually feel comfortable and adopt this grasp position all the time. Using a pencil grip helps some children to position their fingers in a tripod grasp on the pencil. Pencil grips are discussed in more detail on page 166.

Occupational therapists use a variety of techniques to help children remember how to hold their pencils. For example, two rubber bands or hair elastics can go around the wrist, then cross and go over the pencil, to hold it resting between the thumb and index finger.

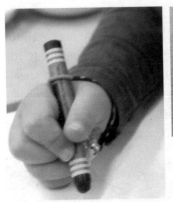

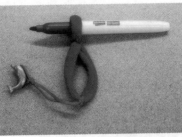

Two hair elastics are looped together, one with a hair bobble. This loop goes over the wrist, with the hair bobble in the palm, to be held by the ring and baby fingers in the palm (hand stability). The other loop goes over the pencil, which naturally holds the pencil in position.

If you look around a regular elementary school classroom, you will see children using different variations of the tripod grasp when printing and writing. A child does not have to hold the pencil in a perfect tripod grasp to be functional in printing and writing. Don't worry if your child doesn't hold the pencil in a perfect dynamic tripod grasp by first grade! Children need time and practice.

All of the ability areas already outlined in this book contribute to a child's ability to master fine control of the pencil for printing, and, eventually, cursive writing. These are very precise skills that many children, with or without Down syndrome, find a challenge.

Children Who Resist Holding Pencils

Some children with Down syndrome do not like to hold anything in their hands. This may not be recognized as a challenge until the child enters school, where he is expected to hold crayons and pencils, scissors, and paintbrushes. This child often holds things by his fingertips to avoid holding them in his palm. If the child demonstrates other avoidance behaviors (not exploring with his hands, not wanting to touch or hold anything, avoiding all sensory play) he may be overly sensitive to touch. Sensory over-responsiveness can lead to these types of behaviors. Strategies for helping a child deal with sensory over-responsiveness—in this case, hypersensitivity to touch in the hands—are discussed in Chapter 11.

Helping Your Child Get Ready to Learn Printing

Preprinting Skills

At first, young preschool children experiment with colors and strokes on the paper that usually do not look like anything in particular. They are experimenting with their ability to direct their hands, and the end result doesn't really matter. Children at this stage benefit from lots of opportunities to experiment, such as painting or drawing on paper at an easel, on a paper or memo board on the fridge, on a blackboard, or on a large paper taped to a table or floor.

At this stage some parents find artwork on their walls! Set up a place for your child that is always available, and clearly let him know that it is acceptable to draw or paint there, but not on the walls, furniture, etc. It is best to keep the supplies handy and available. Usually a child spends only a few minutes at a time at these activities, which only becomes frustrating for the parent who takes everything out and then has to put it all away again a few minutes later.

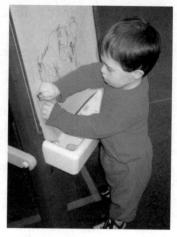

I suggest often placing the paper up at eye level (on an easel or blackboard, or taped to the fridge) for several reasons. First, positioning the activity so that the hands come up in front of the eyes is beneficial for eye-hand coordination when your child is first learning how to direct a pencil on paper. Second, it helps the continued development of shoulder stability and wrist positioning. Your child begins using large strokes, with movements of his whole arm.

Drawing at an easel can help develop eye-hand coordination and shoulder stability.

If using paper on a table or floor, you can tape it down so it doesn't move around. When your child has developed more control, he will be able to stabilize the paper with his other hand.

This is the developmental progression for printing and coloring abilities:

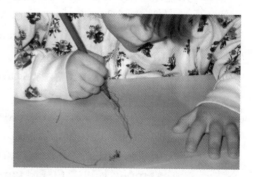

The nondominant hand should automatically hold the paper steady in paper and pencil tasks.

1. Scribbling: making random marks on the paper;
2. Scribbling strokes oriented in a direction (vertical/ horizontal/diagonal);
3. Separate strokes: vertical and horizontal lines;
4. Circles: continuous circular strokes;
5. Strokes becoming more controlled and precise (e.g., a closed circle);
6. Simple combination of circles, lines, and dots (e.g., a variety of forms on the page or combining vertical and horizontal lines to make a cross);

7. Coloring without much regard for the form on the page; may use primarily one color;

8. Diagonal lines;

9. Strokes with changes of direction (e.g., corners);

10. Coloring with some attention to the form, but unable to stay inside the lines and color not always appropriate;

11. Simple shapes (e.g., square, triangle);

12. Simple representational pictures (e.g., face, person, sun, tree, rainbow);

13. Coloring with more attention to detail of the form, attempts to stay inside the lines, some attention to appropriate color;

14. First letters: usually children first learn to print their own names in capital (uppercase) letters. Reversal of letters and numbers is common initially;

15. Coloring with attention to the detail of the picture, choosing appropriate colors; more success at staying in the lines.

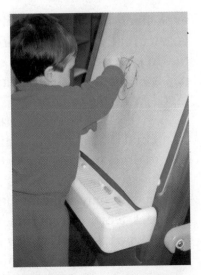

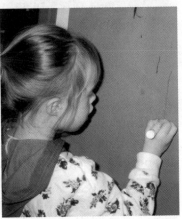

Preprinting skills: lines and circles prepare children to print letters and to draw representational pictures.

16. Letters: children are usually taught to print upper case letters first, then lower case. In my experience, letters with simple linear combinations are easier to learn to print at first. Letters that combine curves, lines, and diagonals are the most difficult initially. For example, I, L, T, O, E, H are easier to learn to print than R, S, M, N, B, W, K, Y.

The Preprinting Developmental Chart outlines the stages of visual motor development, the developmental skills that are emerging concurrently, and activity suggestions for reinforcing these emerging skills.

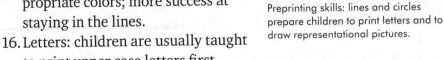

Preprinting Developmental Chart

Stage & Description	Developmental Skills	Suggested Activities for Preprinting Preparation
1. mouthing crayon, crinkling paper 2. banging crayon on paper 3. scribbles randomly, watches others	Child: • takes things in-out; on/off • attends to books • holds crayon in palmar grasp • sits independently • attends to others when they draw • picks up using thumb • points to objects	• sensory play & hand rhymes for sensory awareness • point to pictures in books • provide exploration with crayons, markers, etc. • balance activities with free-arm movement • cause-effect play • encourage thumb use in picking up objects
4. (a) scribbles spontaneously in vertical direction, watching direction of movement of crayon on paper (b) scribbles spontaneously in horizontal direction 5. scribbles spontaneously in circular direction	• develops better control with hands (can stack a few blocks, insert pegs) • begins to match (single shape) • begins to join in with actions in simple familiar songs (e.g., "Wheels on the Bus") • understands up/down • opposes thumb to index for small objects (pincer) • begins to identify body parts • often switches hands during visual motor play	• tabletop activites (puzzles, Duplo, blocks): learns about form in space, and language used in teaching printing, such as up, down or on top • encourage imitation in action songs and, if appropriate, simple signs • finger feeding for pincer grasp • begin spoon feeding for control of wrist • sensory visual motor play; e.g., finger painting, paint with brush, chalk, coloring
6. (a) imitates a vertical & horizontal direction (b) imitates a circular scribble direction 7. (a) imitates vertical & horizontal lines (b) imitates a circular line	• holds crayon in palm with fingers extended, or in crude tripod grasp • completes simple sorting & puzzle activities • picks up scissors, often with 2 hands; attempts to snip • understands 1–2-part directions • actively participates in action songs/signing	• use different surfaces for visual motor play (easel, table, floor) • encourage visual discrimination skills in sorting activities • offer child scissors (loop or squeeze type initially) • sensory play for hand strengthening (play dough, dry sensory for scooping, etc.) • finger songs/rhymes

8. copies vertical & horizontal line 9. (a) copies circle (b) imitates a cross 10. imitates a right/left diagonal	• adds lines, circles, and dots spontaneously to drawings • understands up/down, on/off, in/out • uses touch to identify and manipulate objects • engages in pretend play • snips with scissors (often thumb down) • usually a dominant hand is becoming evident • recognizes some letters • draws simple representational pictures	• imitation in visual motor and game activities • encourage tripod grasp if necessary by providing small pieces of crayon/chalk • manipulative play that strengthens grasping patterns (e.g., stringing beads, foam puzzles, Duplo) • snip play dough, straws, heavy paper (e.g., paint chips, cards) • introduce concrete pre-printing materials, such as the wood pieces in Handwriting without Tears program • complementary worksheets for pencil control (such as at the end of this book) • play simple games on personal electronic device (tablet) or computer
11. copies a right/left diagonal 12. copies a square 13. copies a left/right diagonal 14. copies an X; imitates a triangle 15. copies a triangle	• adds shapes to drawings • attempts to imitate some letters (usually name) • names some letters • understands simple directionality (top to bottom, left to right) • cuts with continuous snips • uses a tripod grasp • colors with more attention to the detail of the picture	• multisensory visual motor activities, such as Magna Doodle, chalk on carpet, finger in sand, etc. • cut along progressively longer lines on heavy paper; add corners and curves when ready • use mouse to make choices on computer • introduce printing program

Stages revised from: Dunn Klein, Marsha. *Pre-Writing Skills*. San Antonio, TX: Therapy Skill Builders, 1990.

Determining Your Child's Readiness for Preprinting Activities

When your child is ready to participate in preprinting activities, he will show these signs:

■ show an interest in toys and manipulative materials beyond banging, throwing, and mouthing them;

- be able to follow simple, one-step instructions (e.g., "hands up");
- watch others;
- make some attempt to imitate;
- have an interest in scribbling and marking on paper.

Helping Your Child Develop Preprinting Concepts

Based on the developmental sequence described above, here are some ideas that I have used in a preprinting program in an inclusive nursery school setting. These activities introduce the basic perceptual concepts involved in printing letters. The concepts that are introduced and reinforced through fun movement and rhythmic games are the following, which are explained in detail below:

- spatial attention and localization: pointing, touching target with marker ("targeting");
- up/down;
- scribbling: getting a "feel" for paper and crayon/marker;
- vertical orientation: standing up tall;
- "top": starting at the top; going from top to bottom;
- horizontal orientation: lying down; "sleeping line";
- same/different;
- left to right;
- top; middle; bottom;
- circles;
- start and stop;
- combining lines: cross.

Spatial Attention and Localization: Your child learns how to focus his visual attention on a specific item. This is necessary in order to be able to imitate or copy a printed letter when learning to print. This skill begins very early, when you are pointing to and naming objects for your child. When your child begins to point himself, you will reinforce his visual attention by also pointing at and naming the object. For example, "Ball. That's a ball. Do you want the ball?" Pointing is very important, as it helps your child direct his visual attention to an object and brings your attention to it as well.

Next, you and your child point to specific people or things in photos and books. Naming and developing little conversations around what your child's visual attention is focused on reinforces his ability to zero in on one part of the picture or photo at a time.

From pointing, you progress to targeting one object on the page or picture and using a marker to indicate it. For example, in a simple coloring book, your child can put his crayon or marker on Barney to begin coloring, thus directing his hand to one particular spot on the page that he is visually focused on. As he gets better at this, he can target increasingly smaller details, such as Barney's mouth, eyes, etc.

At this stage, your child's grasp of the marker is not as important as being able to localize and direct his hand to a particular spot. He can use any kind of writing tool: marker, crayon, chalk, paint-brush, etc. Other activity suggestions for this skill include the following:

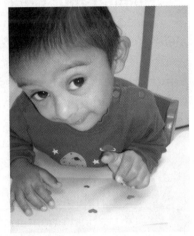

Targeting stickers on a paper develops eye-hand coordination.

- Scatter stickers randomly on a large paper; your child "zooms" in (like an airplane) to each sticker, first with his finger, then with a crayon or marker.
- Jan Olsen, in her *Handwriting without Tears* program, has developed a preschool workbook that devotes several pages to this targeting and visual attention skill (59; also see Resources).

Up/Down: Your baby learns that when he lifts up his arms to be picked up, you pick him up. Simply saying the words *up* and *down* when you pick him up and put him down introduces the language long before your child hears the words in relation to paper-and-pencil activities. Simple games such as bouncing up and down on your knee, tossing up and down in the air, and bouncing up and down to the rhyme "The Grand Old Duke of York" help your child feel what *up* and *down* mean spatially.

"Hands up. Hands down" is a transition chant we use at the nursery school to help the children stop what they are doing and make the transition to the next part of the day. "Up" and "down" are often among the first words we hear a child say at nursery school. Up and down become fascinating when the child learns to go up and down stairs, and parents know how many times a child will repeat going up and down over and over again! He is practicing his gross motor skills, and also feeling the movement of up and down in space.

Here are some other activity suggestions for preschool-aged children:

- Reach way up in standing (such as trying to reach a hanging stream-er or balloon) and then crouch down low to touch the ground.
- Jump up high, then down low.
- Climb up on a platform and jump down.
- At a large blackboard or easel, direct the chalk/paintbrush up and down.

Scribbling: Scribbling is an important first step in the visual motor skills of coloring and printing. All children scribble before they learn to isolate strokes on a paper. Even though it doesn't look like much, your child is developing control of arm and hand movements and visual attention through scribbling. It is exciting to be able to mark up a paper with color by scribbling!

Initially, scribbling is very random, but as your child develops, you will notice that the scribbling will assume definite directional orientation, such as vertical scribble vs. circular or horizontal scribble. This is the precursor to developing directional strokes. Children usually first color with scribbles, with gradually more and more localization to the picture on the page. At first, many children use large arm movements without good control. They need to use large pieces of paper if you want to avoid marks on the floor, table, or wall. Gradually, your child will be able to refine his arm movements to keep his scribble to a smaller space.

Vertical Orientation: Most printed letters have one or more lines with vertical orientation. You can use games and activities to reinforce your child's recognition of "vertical" long before he is ready to print:

- Draw a vertical line down your child's back (starting at the top) with your finger, small brush, small toy, etc., so he feels "vertical."
- Place long felt strips vertically on a felt board.
- Move streamers up and down through the air.
- Tape vertical strips of paper on the wall as a measure of your child's height.
- Place a rectangular block in a vertical orientation; comment that the block is "standing up tall."
- Place wooden sticks with Velcro on the back to a felt or carpet board in a vertical orientation (the sticks are "standing up tall"). The wooden sticks I use in these activities are from Jan Olsen's *Handwriting without Tears* program. Other sticks could be used (such as popsicle sticks) to teach the same concept.

Top: *Top* is an important word for children to understand in a motor context before they begin to learn to print, as we begin printing many letters at the top and move the pencil down. Here are some games and activities to reinforce this concept:

- Have your child put something on *top* of his head (sometimes looking in the mirror can help).
- Use wooden sticks with Velcro on the back and have your child stick them in a vertical orientation on a felt board. He then places a sticker at the *top* of the stick.

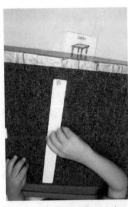

The child places the stick in the vertical orientation.

- Have your child orient a tall narrow block into a vertical ("standing up") position; then place a small toy on *top*.
- Hang a large piece of paper on the wall for drawing vertical lines. A visual cue can be placed along the top to remind your child to start drawing his line at the *top*.
- Let your child draw hair on *top* of a stick figure drawing on the wall.
- Any activity in which your child places something on top will help him understand this concept.

Horizontal Orientation: Again, you will notice your child's scribbling becoming more differentiated, sometimes being more horizontal, sometimes more vertical, sometimes more circular. There are many ways that the horizontal orientation can be reinforced. Here are a few ideas:

- Draw a horizontal "sleeping" line across your child's back.
- Have your child place long blocks end to end to make a long horizontal block path. Then he can walk along the path.
- A rectangular block can be placed lying down or "sleeping."

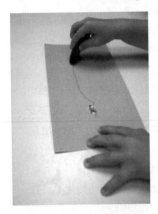

Joining dots involves targeting left to right, start/stop, and horizontal concepts.

- Lie down on the floor ("sleeping"). Sometimes children can understand the words "lying down" or "sleeping" in relation to a horizontal line more easily than the word "across," which gets confusing when drawing a "cross."
- Wooden sticks with Velcro on the back can be placed on the felt board in a horizontal position.
- Play with streamers, moving the arm back and forth in a horizontal direction.
- Place a long narrow strip of paper horizontally on the floor or wall; your child can stroke lines in a horizontal direction across the strip.
- Name cards are horizontal. Children can stick their name cards on a board.

Same/Different: As your child participates in the above activities, you will be able to tell if he recognizes the difference between vertical and horizontal. To reinforce *same,* use the word to describe anything your child does in imitation. For example, if you are playing with rectangular blocks, placing them vertically "up tall," point out that they are standing up the *same* way.

Matching is a concept that children develop as they understand that objects are "the same" or "different." During the preschool or early school years, children learn to match colors that are the same, shapes that are the same, pictures that are the same, etc. This is a visual discrimination and cognitive ability that will develop when your child is ready. If your child has this understanding, you can reinforce it in relation to visual motor skills with these activities:

- taking turns placing felt strips the same way on a board (e.g., all horizontally);
- taking turns imitating each other's strokes on paper;
- matching letters and numbers;
- differentiating *big/little*: use the language that your child is used to hearing (*big/little* or *large/small*). (Matching and sorting by size introduces the concept that he will need to form big vs. little strokes in printing letters);
- finding two pictures/shapes on the page that are the same.

Left to Right: In English, reading and writing move across the page from left to right. Children eventually need to learn to print and read from left to right across the page. Also, most letters are printed starting with the left stroke and then doing the right stroke. It is normal for children to make strokes and do activities in both directions, and I am not suggesting that you must *always* move from left to right. Children who are left-handed will often draw horizontal lines from right to left initially, as this is more natural for them. However, there are ways to help your child recognize the left-to-right orientation for reading and writing in our culture:

- When you are reading to your child, point to the words on the page.
- Let him watch as you print his name on his drawings and paintings.
- Slide his finger across his name card as you say or spell out his name.

Bottom/Middle: As your child begins to make vertical strokes, talk about starting at the top and going down to the bottom. Just as your child placed a sticker at the top of the vertical wooden piece, he can place a sticker at the bottom. As he begins to learn to print, if the concept of starting at the top is reinforced, the idea of *bottom* will develop naturally. *Middle* is a more abstract concept that will probably develop later than *top* and *down*.

Middle comes into play when forming letters such as E, H, F, P, A, B, R, where a horizontal or curve stroke starts/stops at the middle of the vertical stroke. We can introduce *middle* through some of these games and activities:

- Run to the middle of the room (with a mark on the floor).
- Step into a hoop and pull it up to the middle of your body (stomach); everyone can try to do the hula!

- Place a rubber band tightly around the middle of the wooden stick; your children can roll it up to the top, back to the middle, down to the bottom, back to the middle.
- Play "monkey in the middle": one person stands in the center between two or more people playing catch and tries to intercept the ball; when he does so, the person whose throw was caught then becomes the "monkey in the middle."
- Place a sticker in the middle of a vertically oriented wooden stick or a long vertical strip of paper on the wall.

Circles: Children scribble in a circular direction early in their visual motor development. It can be another one to two years, however, before they draw a closed, single circle. At this early stage of visual motor development, introducing circles'helps them to discriminate between straight and circular objects and strokes on paper. Some circle activities include the following:

- Peek through small rings or discs with holes.
- Put bracelets/rings on over hands and feet.
- Crawl/step through hoops.
- Crawl through a tunnel.
- Place round stickers inside a big circle drawn on a paper.
- Place round stickers on paper; then draw a circle around the sticker.
- Make circular shapes with streamers by moving your arm in a circle.
- Many treats are round circles, such as Cheerios, Froot Loops, and Life Savers; these can be used in creative activities.
- Draw eyes on an incomplete face picture.

Start/Stop: Another concept that children develop is the ability to begin a pencil stroke at a defined spot and to stop at a defined spot. For example, when your child changes from making continuous circular strokes to a single circle that comes back to where he started, he is developing this concept. The same is true for simple shapes. In order to be able to attempt a corner—for a square or triangle, for example—your child has to stop the stroke to change direction. Your child needs to understand these concepts to be able to learn to print letters and numbers. Here are some suggested activities for the concept of start/stop:

- motor activities, such as marching and stopping on command; dancing to music and stopping when the music stops;
- running and stopping to a visual or sound cue;
- music activities with instruments, such as shaking bells in a song and stopping at the end;
- tapping and clapping activities, stopping and starting on cue.

When your child understands the concept of *start/stop* through these types of motor activities, visual motor start/stop activities can be introduced, such as:

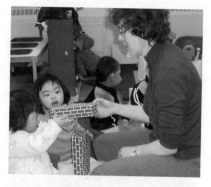

- starting a vertical or horizontal line on a green dot, stopping at the red dot;
- matching worksheets, where the child draws a line to join the two pictures that are the same;
- dot-to-dot activities to reinforce the idea of a definite start/stop point, and number and letter sequencing;
- visual motor worksheets (see Appendix 1);
- mazes, which can help a child learn to begin a stroke and then stop and change direction. Look for simple mazes at this early stage of visual motor development, with a simple path that clearly indicates the starting and finishing points, with one or two changes of direction.

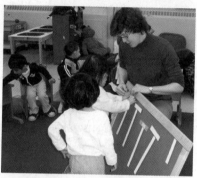

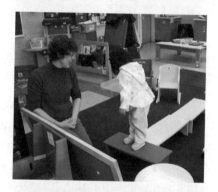

Combining Lines (e.g., Cross): Typically developing children begin to combine a single vertical and horizontal line to form a cross around the age of three. At this stage, we are introducing the concept of combining lines that go in different directions and encouraging imitation of these movements in motor activities.

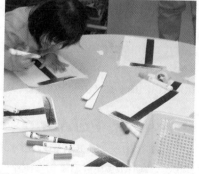

- Trace two long blocks in a cross pattern on a paper. You place one block on the pattern and have your child place the other block in the other direction to form the cross. If you demonstrate and then place the block

This sequence shows some of the activities used in a preschool preprinting group: exploring the letter T using blocks; the *Handwriting without Tears* wooden pieces; a gross motor activity using benches; and finally, tracing T on paper.

Learning the sequence of forming the letter with the wood pieces helps prepare children for learning the sequence of printing the letter.

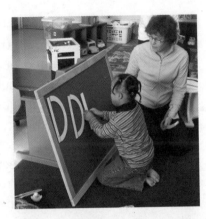

in your child's hands in the proper orientation, he will almost always place it down to form a cross, thus experiencing success. This is your starting point! Next time, you can demonstrate placing both blocks down to form the cross.

■ Have your child hold one wooden stick in each hand and tap them together. Get him tapping in rhythm ("tap, tap, tap… and stop"), stopping with the sticks crossed over each other, so he can experience making a cross with two sticks.

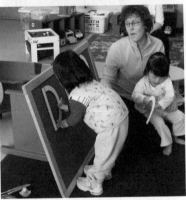

■ Make a cross on the floor with low benches or balance beams and walk along it.

■ Place felt strips on a felt board in a cross pattern, starting with the vertical strip.

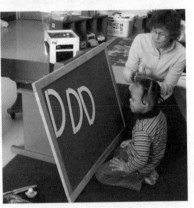

At this stage, children usually combine a variety of strokes and forms on paper. They certainly should be encouraged to do this! They will put circles and lines together (sun, stick person, animals), lines going in different directions (house, car), and usually will add dots. Some demonstration by adults is okay, but it is important that your child experiment and discover for himself how these combinations can represent something, not that he can copy your drawing.

Drawing, Painting, and Coloring

Drawing is the child's first experience of expressing a thought or idea on paper. You may want to show your child how combining forms on paper can represent something in real life. For example, a circle with lines coming out all around represents a sun. Experiment together to give your child more ideas. Representing ideas on paper with pictures may help prepare your child for representing ideas and information on paper with words.

As children commonly include a person or people in their drawings, there are actually developmental norms for this. The face is first to be represented, with simple circular or linear features for the eyes, nose, and mouth. When children begin to represent the body, it is usually as a "stick person," with a line or circle for the body, and single lines representing the arms and legs. As children get older, they add more dimension and shape to the body and limbs, and more detail to the facial features.

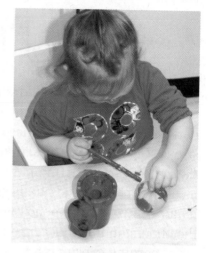

When your child begins to learn to color in pictures, he will use large arm movements across the page to fill in the spaces. Often there isn't much regard for color choice, and he may even use only one color. You may see abrupt changes of direction of the crayon stroke: he may begin with a vertical arm movement and then switch to a horizontal movement. As your child matures, he will attempt to define different parts of the picture by using different colors, but he won't yet be able to stay in the lines. As he gradually develops stability at the shoulder, elbow, and wrist and uses the

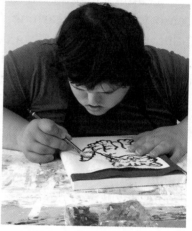

small joints of the hand for movement of the crayon, his coloring will become more refined. His attempts at staying in the lines will be more successful, and he will be able to contour his strokes to the outline of the picture. Color choice usually becomes more varied and appropriate.

Painting provides a vivid sensory experience that children of all ages love. The texture and feel of the paint on the end of the brush gives sensory feedback, and sometimes the strokes that a child makes with a paintbrush are more deliberate and controlled than when using other coloring tools. As painting is often done at an easel, the eye-hand coordination, wrist position, and grasp development is enhanced. Many youth and adults who have Down syndrome continue to express themselves creatively through painting, each with their own unique style.

Appendix 1 has visual motor worksheets that I have developed to use with Sarah and other children. These can be used as a fun exercise to improve refinement of pencil strokes, from preprinting to cursive writing stages.

Printing

Developing the ability to direct a pencil on paper in preprinting practice prepares children to learn to print letters. The preprinting activities previously described help your child to learn how to form the "parts" of the letters. These activities give him lots of practice making lines, circular strokes (going in both directions), and diagonals. He also comes to understand the concept of a starting point and a stopping point, and has an idea of the meaning of letters and numbers. The next step is for your child to integrate his motor control with a pencil with his visual perceptual development; that is, the understanding that certain forms represent a concept (a letter or number).

Learning to print is a complex process involving the integration of visual, sensory, and motor learning. All children benefit from watching someone else print the letter, so they can observe the movements involved. Over time, the movements become automatic as the pathways are established in the brain. If the child learns incorrect letter formation due to lack of models and coaching, it will be more difficult to "undo" the learned movement patterns and reteach correct formation. If the child is expected to learn to print before he is developmentally ready, he may develop incorrect patterns of letter formation to compensate for the lack of visual motor foundation skills. If you focus on building strong preprinting foundation skills for your child with Down syndrome, it will provide the groundwork for learning to print *when he is ready*.

Determining Your Child's Readiness for Printing

So when is he ready? These are some of the questions I would consider when deciding if a child is ready to learn to print:

1. Can the child hold a writing tool, preferably a pencil? The development of pencil grasp was discussed earlier in this chapter. Printing requires control of small movements in the hands. If a child is using a palmar grasp, he is not usually ready to learn to print. However, there are exceptions to this, as some children have developed the perceptual and cognitive readiness for printing but are delayed in fine motor control. For most children, holding a pencil in an immature tripod grasp is the starting point for learning the pencil control necessary to print functionally in workbooks and on worksheets.

2. Can the child imitate in visual motor activities? For example, if you draw a horizontal line, can he imitate it? Can he imitate more

complex patterns, such as a cross, closed circle, diagonal line? If the child is not yet able to imitate some of the preprinting strokes, he is probably not ready to learn to print. I usually begin with the easiest upper case letters before a child can consistently copy or even imitate diagonals and a square. There are differences of opinion on this.

3. Does the child display an interest in and attention to visual motor activities? Is he motivated to participate in drawing with markers and crayons, coloring, painting, and using a pencil? If motivated, he is more likely to have the attention necessary to learn to print.

4. Does the child spontaneously draw some or all of the preprinting strokes, such as directional lines, circles, dots, zigzags, and combinations of these? In other words, does he initiate some of these strokes himself when painting, coloring, etc., without any adult direction?

5. Does the child have the body stability to sit in a chair at a table and direct the movement of his hand with the pencil?

6. Does the child have the cognitive level to understand the meaning of printing? If the child understands that letters form words that symbolize objects and people, he will be much more motivated to participate in a printing program. Otherwise, it becomes a meaningless fine motor exercise. Sound-letter recognition (understanding the sounds each letter can make) will develop over time, while the child is learning to read and print.

Printing His Name

Usually the first word that children learn to print is their name. As mentioned above, your child will be motivated to print if it has meaning for him.

Profile: Sarah

At five years old, Sarah was having difficulty mastering diagonal lines. I found that using a calendar helped. Every day she would take the calendar down from the bulletin board, removing the thumb tack, and would put an x through the date. I showed her how to start in the top corner and go across to the opposite corner. We started doing only one line, from the top left corner to the bottom right. When she was able to do that consistently, we added the other diagonal line from the bottom left to the top right corners. Putting the calendar back up on the bulletin board with the thumb tack helped strengthen her pincer grasp. After doing this for a couple of months, she was able to make diagonal lines anywhere. This activity also helped reinforce the days of the week, number recognition, and the months of the year.

First your child recognizes the sound of his name, later he recognizes his printed name, and then he learns to print it himself. Often, even if the child is not really ready to begin a *printing program* as such, he will be taught how to print his name. This is fine, as usually the child is motivated and is pleased with any attempts, even if they aren't exactly correct.

Positioning

Positioning for printing is very important. It helps provide the stability that is one of the building blocks for developing pencil control. According to some researchers, however, many children with Down syndrome lack this stability. In observing children with Down syndrome doing handwriting activities, the researchers noted that most assumed a slouched posture after a short period of time, and some "hitched" the shoulder of their writing arm in an attempt to stabilize (5).

When your child has developed the early preprinting skills on larger paper at an easel or similar setup, and he is ready to begin working at a desk or table, keep in mind the following positioning considerations:

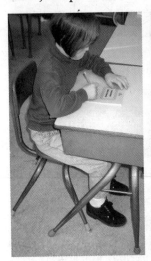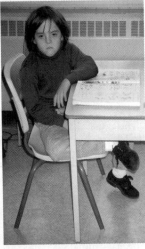

It is important for your child to have a comfortable table or desk to work at. The desk and chair on the left are the right height. Those on the right are too high. When the chair is too high, the child may twist in the chair in order to touch the floor with a foot.

1. The chair and desk should be the right size for your child. Although this seems basic, it is often overlooked. Knees should be in line with hips, or slightly higher, but not lower, and feet flat on the floor, directly under the knees. If the available chair is too high, place a sturdy footstool under the feet. Elbows should rest comfortably on the desk, without the shoulders being elevated (desk is too high), or hunched (desk is too low).

2. Sometimes children with lower muscle tone find it difficult to sit up straight for long periods at a desk, even with correct desk size, and end up leaning their head down on their other arm while they work. Sometimes working on a slanted surface, something like a drafting table or slanted writing board, can help. I have used an empty binder, two inches wide or more at the spine, on the desk, slanting up away from the child. When I used this with

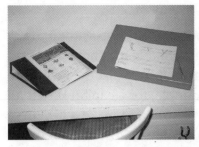

A slanted writing table can help some children with low muscle tone to keep an upright sitting posture when printing. A binder can also be used.

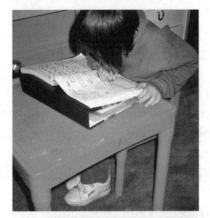

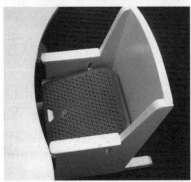

Movin' Sit cushion

Sarah, she was better able to maintain an upright sitting posture while printing, and didn't put her face down as close to her work. Another strategy for children with low tone who tire quickly is to offer a variety of printing positions and techniques. Doing some work at the computer, some at the desk, some at an easel or the blackboard, some on the floor, each for shorter periods, may enable them to complete more written work.

3. Consider your child's desk position in the classroom or at home. Factors such as lighting, position relative to the teacher, and nearby distractions will all affect how your child works at the desk.

4. Providing a cushion that allows for some movement and sensory input can help activate the muscles for maintaining an upright position. Here are some suggestions:

   - Try placing a small beach ball with a tiny bit of air in it on your child's chair, just enough to allow for a little bit of movement input.
   - Put a "Movin' Sit" or Disc 'O' Sit cushion on his chair (see Resources).
   - Have your child sit on a therapy ball with feet on the floor. Therapy balls can be purchased with a base to prevent them from rolling around (see Flaghouse and Sammon-Preston in Resources). A ball can be used at a desk instead of a chair.

Printing Sequence

Children with Down syndrome usually learn to print by following the sequence outlined here:

1. Imitating,
2. tracing and copying,
3. printing independently, and
4. printing on lines.

Imitating

Your child watches you make the letter and then either traces on top of yours, or makes his own. By watching you, your child learns how the letter is formed and how to break it down into its parts. It may also be helpful to describe what you are doing as you do it. For example, for a capital D, "First I draw a straight line down; then I jump back to the top and make a big curve around to the bottom." Talking your child through it may be more successful than helping him hand over hand. By talking through it, you give your child another sensory message (auditory) to help him remember. You also give him a little more independence than with hand-over-hand assistance.

Tracing and Copying

Tracing should be done after the child has had the opportunity to imitate and to watch someone form the letter. When tracing, he makes his strokes directly over the model. In copying, the model is there for him to see, but he has to remember how to make it. He has to remember the process of breaking down the letter into its parts and putting them together. This is obviously harder than imitating. Also, copying from the blackboard is harder than copying from a sample right in front of him, such as an alphabet strip on his desk.

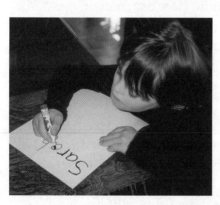

Some markers change the underlying color when traced. When your child traces over your printing with his marker, the color changes, or an interesting effect appears. This makes tracing more motivating for many children.

I do not recommend tracing as the first step in teaching a child to print. All children will learn better printing habits if they are taught how to form the letters and then have supervised printing practice, during which they use the correct patterns. If a child is given worksheets to trace before he knows how the letters are formed, he is likely to be inconsistent in the letter pattern. This will make it more difficult for him to progress to independent printing. Tracing can be one method used to practice printing once your child knows how to form the letters correctly.

Copying is often used with children with Down syndrome in the classroom. Usually the educational assistant or teacher prints out the lesson and the child copies it underneath. This is called "underwriting." Again, this should only be used once the child has learned how to print well enough that he can form the letters automatically. Adults must remember to leave extra space between words so that the child, whose printing is usually larger, can continue to copy directly underneath the adult's words. In the higher grades, when there are large amounts of written work in a day, the child with Down syndrome may be copying many pages of printing. The challenge is to keep this written work meaningful for the child, so that he is reading and understanding the content as well as copying it. The goals in copying skills are the following:

1. looking at each letter and copying them one by one;
2. looking at a whole word and copying it without having to glance back up at it;
3. looking at a short sentence and copying it without repeatedly glancing up at it.

A child's ability to progress through these stages depends largely on literacy development, rather than on fine motor skills.

Printing Independently

This is the next stage of learning how to print letters and numbers. Your child must be able to recall the visual image of the letter and remember how to direct his hand to reproduce this on the page.

Thinking up imaginative anecdotes about particularly tricky letters or numbers may help your child remember how to form them. The cues and anecdotes you make up will be best remembered if they are interesting for your child. For example, in order to help Sarah remember how to form the number five, I used this visual image: there is a little man (straight line down) with a big round tummy (semicircle) and a hat (horizontal line on top). When she couldn't remember how to form a five, reminding her about the little man helped her remember how to get started.

Some letters and numbers are easily confused because the pattern is similar except for the initial starting direction. For quite a long time, Sarah printed her name beginning with an S or a 3, depending on which way her pencil began to move! Other letters that are easily confused are M & W, b & d, p & q, n & u. If your child has learned the pattern for each letter, he will probably have less trouble with reversals and inversions. For example, *b* begins with a vertical line down, and can be learned at the same time as the other letters that begin in the same way (h, k, l, p). If *d* is also taught by beginning with the vertical line down, it may cause confusion. Instead, it can be taught by beginning with the curved stroke, at the same time as the other letters that begin that way (a, g, q). At the end of this chapter, I give one suggested way of grouping lowercase letters for learning to print. Other educators and therapists may use similar groupings when teaching printing.

When your child is ready to practice printing letters, there are many commercially available workbooks that provide direction and practice, some with wipe-off pages. Most of these books have arrows that show the child which direction the line or curve should go. However, your child with Down syndrome may have difficulty following arrows. Without supervision, he may randomly attempt to trace and copy the letters. It is generally thought to be best for the child to learn to print with consistent direction of his strokes (59). Until your child is consistently printing letters in the right direction, it may be best to continue with imitating (so he can see how you form the letter) and supervised copying. Once he has established the patterns of movement for printing the letters, he could use the printing workbooks for more practice. The book *Handwriting without Tears,* by Jan Z. Olsen, describes one program for teaching printing and cursive writing that is successful for many children. Workbooks are included in the program (59).

Here are some more examples of verbal cues to give your child to help him remember the visual image of the letter or number, and how to initiate the printing sequence. These are only a few examples. What works for your child will depend partly on his interests. If he particularly likes trains, for example, you can talk about "n" being a single train tunnel, "m" being a

Alternatives to Paper and Pencil

During these first three stages of printing development, offering a variety of ways to practice may help keep your child motivated and will keep it fun. Using a multisensory approach can help some children learn letter shapes more easily. Here are some ideas:

- finger painting letters, numbers, and shapes
- coloring apps, in which a finger is used to apply color to pictures
- learning-to-print apps, which guide the child to use a finger to trace letters
- drawing in sand with a stick
- sidewalk chalk
- Magna Doodle
- colorful chalk for a blackboard
- paintbrush dipped in water: make letters, etc. on outside walls, fences, etc.
- drawing with a finger in flour; powder; dry Kool-Aid or Jell-O mix
- making letters, etc., with cooked spaghetti noodles;
- making letters, etc., with "Wikki Stix" (colorful string dipped in wax);
- rolling out a snake of play dough and forming a letter. (The last three activities will be easier initially if your child makes his letter on top of a large printed letter.)

double tunnel, etc. Even with this type of cuing, learning to print takes lots of time and practice.

- h: a tall line with a hump;
- r: a small line with a roof;
- s: a slithery snake;
- w: choppy waves;
- j: a fishing line and hook going down into the water.

Printing on Lines

Once your child can print letters independently, he will gradually begin to refine his printing to be able to stay on lines, with consistent size and spacing. This stage may be as difficult as learning to print the letters themselves. It is hard enough to remember how to form all the letters while retaining the understanding of the words and sentences being printed, let alone having to worry about staying on the lines! Recognize how challenging this is, and support your child in every attempt to print. If the demands are too great, he might refuse to keep trying.

Here are some strategies that may help your child develop the ability to print on the lines with consistent size:

1. Widely spaced lines should be used initially, as your child's printing will be quite large. You can draw the lines with a ruler on unlined paper.

2. When your child begins to reduce the size of his printed letters, he may benefit from using some specialized paper. Using paper with very dark lines may help direct the printing orientation. Janice Z. Olson, in her book *Handwriting without Tears,* suggests using two lines, a top and bottom line, without the dotted or multicolored lines that some primary workbooks have. Also available in some educational stores is raised-line paper (such as Right-Line Paper, by Pro-Ed), so the child can feel where the line is. If your child doesn't always begin his printing on the left side of the page, you can put a small green dot there to remind him.

3. Another strategy sometimes used is to make boxes on the page for the child to fill in the letters; this helps him learn size and word spacing and to stay on a horizontal line.

4. Leave plenty of space between words if your child is copying under someone else's printing. If there is not enough space between words, his words will run together. Children learning to print always need more space.

5. Underline the space under the word to be copied to give your child a cue as to where to place his word and how to space his copying.

When your child is printing at school and is trying to master all these skills, discuss the type of approach to use with your child's teacher (and occupational therapist, if one is involved). Many children with Down syndrome will learn to print on lines with correct spacing without using specialized paper; it just takes time!

Pencil Pressure

Sometimes a child may have difficulty with the amount of pressure he uses on the pencil. Pressure can be affected by position and posture (pages 160-61), by the type of grasp used and where the pencil is held, by the type of pencil or pen used, and by the child's experience with printing. If too much pressure is used, it may give him a tight, cramped hand, and he may rip the paper. More often, children with Down syndrome use too little pressure, resulting in printing that is very light and wobbly. A heavier lead in the pencil or a felt-tip marker can help the child who uses too little pressure. A weighted pencil (a small weight that slides on and off a regular pencil) may provide more sensory input so the child can use appropriate pressure. A pencil grip or tactile cue can help him hold the pencil with a firmer grasp.

Sometimes a pencil grip is useful for children who hold the pencil too tightly and use too much pressure. A child may hold the pencil too tightly in an attempt to stabilize if he lacks stability in the body and shoulder. If this is the problem, activities as suggested in Chapter 5 will be helpful.

Pencil Grips: Sometimes a special grip on the pencil will help your child place his hand in the right spot and maintain a tripod grasp. There are several types of pencil grips available commercially, including

- Foam grip
- Triangle grip
- Stetco Grip
- Writing Claw
- Grotto Grip
- Start Right Grip
- The Pencil Grip

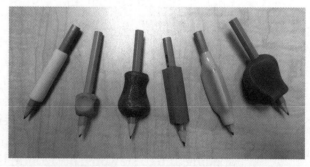

Left to right: foam grip , Stetco Grip, The Pencil Grip, two examples of triangle grips, Grotto Pencil Grip.

I have had the most experience and success with The Pencil Grip and Stetco pencil grips (see Resources).

Pencil grips can be helpful for the child who can achieve a tripod grasp on a pencil when it is placed there for him, but:

1. has difficulty remembering how to position the pencil in his fingers himself,

2. uses the base of the thumb to hold the pencil against the side of his hand (the thumb wrap grasp, or anchoring grasp, described earlier in the chapter), or
3. can't achieve or maintain a tripod grasp on the pencil

However, for some children, pencil grips are more distracting than beneficial. Because the child isn't holding on to the pencil directly, but on to the grip, some control of the pencil movement is lost.

Tactile and Visual Cues: If your child holds the pencil too far up the shaft, his writing hand is completely off the paper, resulting in light pressure and less control. A sticker or pencil grip indicating where the pencil should be held can help your child position the pencil more effectively. Alternately, you can make a mark on your child's hand, between the thumb and index finger, to indicate where the pencil should rest against his hand.

As mentioned previously, you can use a hair elastic band around your child's wrist and pencil to help him maintain the position of the pencil and enable him to use more consistent pencil pressure.

Cursive Writing

Most children learn handwriting (cursive writing) in third or fourth grade. This is too early for most children with Down syndrome. Some of our children may never learn functional cursive writing. They will need to be able to print or write their signature, but may not need to learn more cursive writing skills. What they will need is some relatively efficient way to communicate in written form. This is often a combination of printing and/or cursive writing and computer use.

Cursive writing demands continuous movement of the small joints of the hand, as the letters are formed in a flowing, nonstop motion. There isn't the opportunity to stop after each letter and reposition the hand for the next letter, as in printing. The adjustments of position in the arm as it moves across the page have to be smooth for handwriting to be efficient. The child must also make small adjustments in posture to accommodate his arm movement. For children who have any difficulty with posture, balance, and stability, handwriting will be more of a physical challenge.

Prewriting exercises can be introduced prior to learning to write individual letters. This is a similar approach to the preprinting activities described earlier in this chapter. Prewriting exercises involve repetitive, flowing patterns that help the child gain control of the continuous, joined movements for writing. For example, making a line of joined loops will help your child develop the motion that begins the letters l, k, b, f, e, and h. As in the preprinting activities, it is often helpful to begin doing these patterns at a blackboard or easel, where the child can move his arm freely and make larger letters.

In Appendix 1, I have included some prewriting worksheets that incorporate the five basic patterns found in most written letters. There are also commercially available handwriting workbooks and programs that incorporate pattern practice and letter formation. Some examples are: *Callirobics* (in which the exercises are done to music); *Neurokinesthetic Writing Program* (#3 in Bibliography); *Handwriting without Tears* (#59 in Bibliography). See the Resources section at the back of the book for sources of handwriting programs.

As with printing, your child may be taught cursive handwriting following the D'Nealian or Zaner-Bloser methods. I don't feel that there is any right or wrong method of teaching handwriting. What is most important is that the child learn *how* to form the letters consistently and efficiently. To do this he must be shown and taught the correct way, otherwise he will devise his own method that will likely not lead to cursive writing success in the long term. Sarah did not develop cursive writing that is automatic enough to replace her printing for efficiency. She continues to use printing and keyboarding as her methods of written communication. When she was practicing cursive during her school years, however, it seemed that the *Handwriting without Tears* program was the easiest for her, as it is based on the printed letter.

Your child may be able to learn writing in the same way most children learn: practicing one letter at a time, going through the alphabet in order. Many children, however, benefit from learning the letters in groups with similar formations. For example, in cursive writing, the letters a, c, d, g, o, and q all begin in the same way. Learning this pattern for a group of letters helps many children remember how to form them.

Cursive writing is the culmination of the development of all the areas described throughout this book. Good stability and control in the body, shoulders, and arms; hand stability and dexterity of the small joints of the hand; sensory awareness and memory of the feel of how to form the letters; visual motor control; cognitive ability; and motivation all contribute to the ability to learn cursive writing. Given all these factors that come into play, it is not surprising that many children, not just children with Down syndrome, find the process of learning cursive writing difficult. When setting goals for our children with Down syndrome, we need to consider the amount of time and effort that may need to be put into learning cursive writing. It is realistic to set a goal of cursive writing if it is expected that the child will be able to eventually use cursive writing as a functional skill.

Accommodations & Modifications
for written work

Most students with Down syndrome need a variety of accommodations and modifications to their classwork and homework at school. This is especially the case when it comes to written work.

Accommodations are changes to some aspect of the program to enable your child to cover the same curriculum and have the same learning expectations as typically developing classmates. For example, a student may be able to use word-prediction software to complete a written assignment rather than writing it out by hand.

Modifications are changes to the curriculum and expectations to meet the learning needs of the student. For example, the written expectations for an assignment are at a lower grade level.

Examples of accommodations and modifications for written work output in the classroom throughout the school years may include:

- dictation to a scribe
- fill-in-the-blank, single-word answers
- short-form answers, rather than complete sentences
- communication software or apps to build sentences
- multiple choice rather than essay answers
- dictation to a voice recorder
- speech-to-text software (sometimes called voice-to-text)
- word-prediction software
- additional time to complete written work

Dictation to a Scribe

Dictation to a scribe is an example of an accommodation that is commonly used for students with Down syndrome. The "scribe," usually an educational assistant, sometimes another student, writes down what the child says. For example, in journal writing, the scribe might first write down what the child describes about what he did last evening. Then, the child usually writes underneath, copying the words above. This is considered an accommodation if all students in the class are expected to write a journal entry on the same topic. It is a modification if the student with Down syndrome is writing a journal entry, while the other students are writing reports for a project.

Scribes are also used to write down information dictated or written on the blackboard by the teacher. Again, often the student copies underneath. Scribes can also be used to assist students during testing situations, if the child knows the material and is able to verbalize it but doesn't have the fine motor skill to write it all down.

When printing independently, the child has to think about the content, the spelling of the words, and the construction of the sentence. If printing or writing is not yet fully automatic, the child will also have to think about the formation of the letters, the spacing, etc. If the goal is printing development, he should not always use a scribe, but may have an assistant to verbally help him with spelling and sentence composition. If the goal is spelling, grammar, and content, he should have a scribe to help him organize the fine motor aspect of putting the information down on paper. There is no magic age when a child should stop using a scribe. High school students with Down syndrome may have a peer tutor to assist with taking notes in order to keep up with the information being presented.

Profile: Mark

Seven-year-old Mark is "underwriting" in his journal at school; that is, his educational assistant prints what he dictates, and he copies underneath. As the lines in the small notebooks are too small for him to write on, his assistant draws lines on unlined paper for him to print on. One day, Mark says he wants to try making the lines. Holding the ruler down while drawing a line promotes stability, as he has to hold it steady, and bilateral coordination, as one hand is using pressure to hold the ruler and the other hand is drawing the line. His assistant also encourages him to pick up his pencil with only his dominant hand, without helping to position it with his other hand. This helps him use small movements in his fingers to orient the pencil in his hand to be ready to print.

Computers & Technology

When I began writing the first edition of this book in the mid 1990s, a single desktop computer in the home was becoming the norm for many families. Now, almost twenty years later, most homes and classrooms and many individuals have a variety of devices that are used throughout the day: laptop and desktop computers, smart phones, and tablets or iPads. Computers and technology are such a part of our lives that it is hard to remember what life was like pre-computer. Much of our work, school work, communication, dissemination of knowledge and news, banking, social networking, entertainment, and leisure involves technology.

Our children, teens, and adults who have Down syndrome are as much a part of this technologically interconnected world as anyone. Like everyone, they must not only learn how to use the devices, but how to be safe and maintain privacy doing so. These days a child's first introduction to technology devices is likely in the home, with their parent's phone, tablet, or computer. Many children do seem drawn to technology, and sometimes parents use it as a reward or motivator. In this section I will focus on fine motor access to technology and fine motor skill development with the help of technology.

SMART Technology in the Classroom

The amount and type of technology available for student use in classrooms seems to be widely variable.

Some classrooms have "SMART Board Interactive Whiteboards" or "SMART Table Interactive Learning Centers," which can provide technological interactivity between teacher and students, and among students. Students can easily access programs on the SMART Board and Table simply by touching. The visual and auditory feedback can make learning fun and interactive. SMART Boards connect to the Internet, making it easy to find photos and videos that enhance learning.

SMART technology also enables students to give nonverbal responses by using a device. These features may be helpful for children with Down syndrome, who benefit from a multisensory learning approach, with an emphasis on visuals and a decreased reliance on fine motor skills.

iPads and Tablet Devices

iPads, tablets, and iPods have opened up a world of seemingly endless possibilities for people with disabilities. These mainstream devices, used by people of all ages, can support engagement in learning, communication, organizational skills, social engagement, fine motor skills development, etc. Many parents, educators, and therapists find that apps designed for social, emotional, communication, and behavioral learning are helpful for their children who have Down syndrome.

Communication apps for the iPad, iTouch, and Android devices have been developed for children who have difficulty with verbal communication. There are several advantages of using an app for communication assistance:

- The cost of the device and apps is much more affordable than most of the previously available voice output devices.
- The iPad, iTouch, and other tablets are more mainstream than other communication devices and are not viewed as disability devices. Therefore, even older students do not feel stigmatized when using them.

For some children with disabilities, particularly those who have autism, using a communication app on a tablet as a text-to-speech interface helps them make unprecedented leaps in their communication. Some children who have Down syndrome are also benefitting from touch screen apps that help them to communicate, giving them a "voice" that might be more easily understood by others. A commonly used app is called Proloquo2Go from AssistiveWare; there are others, and anyone interested in communication technology for their child should investigate all options and consult with a speech pathologist who knows your child's needs and abilities.

The availability of apps aimed at supporting child development is overwhelming. Some organizations provide online lists that can help the parent of a child who has Down syndrome sort through the options. Here are a few examples:

- Down Syndrome Daily (www.downsyndromedaily.com)
- DSAQ Guide to Apps (http://www.dsaq.org.au/publications/dsaq-guide-to-apps-2nd-edition)
- BridgingApps (www.bridgingapps.org)
- OTs with APPS & Technology (www.otswithapps.com)

Fine Motor Advantages of Using a Tablet Device

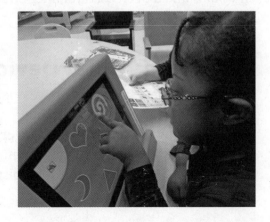

Many children who have Down syndrome have difficulty holding and using a pencil to complete worksheets and other written schoolwork. Touch screen apps provide countless learning opportunities, removing the challenge of paper-and-pencil work. Children can complete activities much more quickly and accurately. Using an app, they are able to focus on the learning task, without significant energy being exerted to execute the fine motor skill required. Unlike a computer, which uses a keyboard and mouse to interface between the hands and the eyes, a touch screen device enables a direct link between the hand and eyes.

Some of the apps specifically designed to improve fine motor skills target some of the following components:

1. Targeting: touching an item on the screen causes a result (e.g., the balloon pops, the squash squishes, etc.). This attention to spatial localization and the ability to direct the hand to the target are important developmental skill. There are many ways to build this skill in a young child, as explained in the section "Helping Your Child Get Ready to Learn Printing." As the child increases in skill, the targets begin to move, with increasing speed and accuracy required. Joining two or more targets with a sliding motion is involved in a dot-to-dot type of activity.

2. Tracing: the child places his finger at the starting point and traces a pattern or letter. There is usually immediate visual and auditory feedback. Some of the patterns are similar to the Stage 1 visual-motor worksheets in Appendix 1, followed by more complex patterns and letters. These tablet activities can be used in conjunction with paper and pencil activities to provide variety and increased feedback.

3. Pinch: some app activities require the child to use a pinching motion between the thumb and first two fingers to achieve the desired result. Development of accurate pinch is also an important developmental skill, as discussed in Chapter 8.

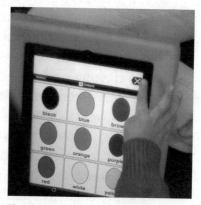

4. Coloring: the child uses his finger to color in a picture and can choose from many colors.

5. Speed and accuracy of eye-hand coordination increases as the level of play increases.

The iPad is protected in a Big Grips frame; the stand brings it up to eye level to support good posture.

Fine Motor Challenges of Using a Tablet Device

One of the main fine motor challenges in using a tablet device I have observed in young children who have Down syndrome is due to hypotonia: their fingers have a tendency to collapse when touching the screen. The child's touch is either ineffective to activate the screen, or the touch is not precise enough. It can be difficult for a young child to learn how long and how hard they should press on the screen with their fingers, which relates to the development of the sense of proprioception. An example of this problem is with the puzzle apps that require a touch-and-slide motion to move puzzle pieces into the correct spots. The child doesn't exert a consistent enough touch through the sliding motion, and the puzzle piece bounces back to its original position, even though the child has made the correct response.

A stylus can be used instead of the finger to touch the screen. However, the stylus is held in the hand in a tripod pencil grasp, which can also be difficult for young children. If the child can't maintain a tripod pencil grasp, an iPad tablet hand pointer, which holds the stylus in the palm, is available (through Bridges; see Resources).

Other challenges include the following:

- A child my inadvertently delete apps if he is using a device in which a sustained touch on the app's icon on the home screen activates the delete option.
- Some young children have a tendency to touch the Home button frequently, which takes them out of the app and back to the home page. Activating "Guided Access" under Accessibility settings on the iPad, which keeps the screen in a single app and controls which features are available, is a solution to this problem. Another solution is to apply a "Bub Cap" over the Home button, which prevents it from being pressed.
- A computer keyboard and mouse is more tactile than a touch screen and therefore provides more sensory feedback than a flat, smooth touch screen. Pressing keyboard keys and moving and clicking a mouse all provide sensory feedback through the fingers and hand and help develop the tactile and proprioceptive senses in the hand. A touch screen provides little sensory feedback. There are no tactile boundaries to define each letter on a touch screen keyboard, for example. A Bluetooth keyboard can be linked to an iPad to overcome this.
- Tablet devices and iPads are fragile and should be protected in rubberized cases. There are now several options available (such as the Big Grips frame and stand).
- If there are a lot of apps on a device, it can be difficult for young children with Down syndrome to locate the one they want. The desktop of a tablet or iPad can be arranged to be less distracting by organizing the apps into folders, thus minimizing the number of icons on the screen.

Accessibility Options

iPads and other tablet devices have accessibility options that provide adaptations for visual, hearing, and physical needs. The Guided Access option on the iPad is very helpful to prevent a child from accidentally exiting an app. A speak selection option will speak aloud text that is highlighted (by double touching at the beginning of the phrase and swiping the finger along to the end of the selected text). This can be helpful for teens and adults who are accessing email and social media, but who need help with reading the text. It requires precise fine motor control to highlight the text to be spoken, and seems to work only on Apple apps and Safari (it doesn't currently seem to work for Facebook).

Computers

The ability to understand how to access technology using a keyboard or touch screen will be a crucial life skill for our children. I hope that all children with Down syndrome will have the opportunity to learn some basic keyboarding skills in school to augment their printing or handwriting skills, and to increase their opportunities for independence in their daily lives.

Computers are used in most elementary and high schools as instructional tools, for data management, and for word processing. In this section, the access to and use of computer hardware and software to assist written communication will be briefly discussed. Decisions about specialized computer options are best made in consultation with a computer expert—either someone within the school or someone from an augmentative communication clinic or program. Companies that sell accessible technology provide consultation and training in the use of the technology. This is a field that is growing all the time, and experts in the field can provide the most up-to-date information about computer access and options.

The information presented here covers these broad areas:
1. keyboard skills;
2. hardware options;
3. accessibility options built into computer operating systems; and
4. software options.

Keyboard Skills

As with printing and writing, positioning is important when using a keyboard: correct work height, back support, feet flat on the floor. When your child's elbows are bent at 90 degrees, the keyboard should be level with or slightly below the hands. The monitor should be at eye level; your child should not have to look up to see the monitor. If your child is doing a lot of typing on a regular basis, I recommend wrist support cushions, which are readily available in office supply stores. These firm wrist support cushions reduce strain and fatigue on the muscles.

Twenty-five years ago, the use of computers with children with Down syndrome in learning and communication programs was not the norm. Laura Meyers, in "Using Computers to Teach Children with Down Syndrome," reported in 1988 that children with Down syndrome often got less frustrated and were more enthusiastic about written communication when they were using a computer than when they were printing or handwriting (52). This statement seems very obvious today, and could be applied to many children, not just those who have Down syndrome. Computers and tablets can be motivating, can help teachers and parents to track change and progress, can help sustain attention through visual and auditory feedback, and can help the child present his knowledge in a more organized, easy-to-read format.

Printing and cursive writing is usually a slow and laborious process for our children due to the difficulties with pencil grasp and visual motor control. Learning the keyboard also takes time for children with Down syndrome, but the physical process may be less difficult than writing. Although touch typing (placing and using all the fingers on the keyboard) is ideal, it is often not practical for children who have fine motor difficulties. In fact, using the "hunt and peck" technique may be more functional for some people. Learning and practicing keyboard skills by doing functional and meaningful computer activities, rather than typing exercises, was cited by teens with fine motor difficulties as the best way to learn keyboarding (56). This could include communicating with their friends through email and Facebook and other chat pages, writing a blog, writing up a shopping list, keeping a daily journal, etc.

In a recent study of computer usage by young individuals with Down syndrome (26), the authors reported that among those families surveyed, 77.5 percent of children between the ages of 5 and 21 use one or both index fingers to type, while 22.5 percent use multiple fingers on one or both hands. Based on their study of expert computer users with Down syndrome, Martin Lazar found that many individuals with Down syndrome can indeed use multiple fingers when typing, when they have had training and sufficient practice. In fact, teens and adults who have Down syndrome continue to use and

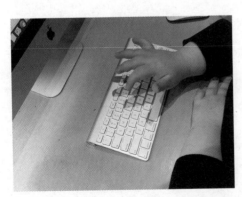
Many people, with and without Down syndrome, use one or two fingers on a keyboard.

develop their fine motor keyboarding skills as they mature, and if given the opportunity, many can perform multiple tasks using a computer and keyboard without modification (41).

There are several software programs to teach keyboarding skills. *Handwriting without Tears* has recently introduced a *Keyboarding without Tears* program. There are many other programs available, and all children going through school should be given the opportunity and training to learn keyboarding and typing, whether that be in a structured typing program or through regular functional use of the computer and keyboard.

Hardware Options

Hardware refers to the physical components of the computer. Hardware options to consider related to writing skills include the following:

- desktop vs. laptop computer
- keyboard options
- mouse options
- touch screen options

Selecting appropriate hardware options can help you minimize language, cognitive, and fine motor difficulties that can interfere with a child's ability to use a computer effectively. In this section, only hardware options related to the fine motor aspect of written communication will be discussed.

Although some school systems have a variety of hardware options available, many do not. You or your child's teachers may have to consult with assistive technology experts, either through a company that sells the hardware or through a hospital or clinic that offers this service. If a trial of a hardware option proves successful, you and the school may want to include it in your child's IEP, if it helps him to meet his educational goals.

Keyboard Options

Usually children with Down syndrome do not need a modified keyboard when they are using a computer or laptop. However, should there be challenges with a regular keyboard, here are some modified options:

- Large key keyboards (such as BigKeys in Qwerty or ABC layout)
- "Zoom Caps" or "Keyboard Seels": high contrast letters that can be stuck on to the keys
- Keyboard overlays/ keyguards for more defined key separation (so that only one key can be hit at a time)
- High contrast/visibility keyboards
- Specialized keyboards (such as Intellikeys by Intellitools), which often have a simplified layout and may require less pressure to press a key

Mice and Alternatives

Using a computer mouse is a good example of an activity that involves using our sensory and perceptual system to guide our fine motor movements. The sensors in our muscles and joints direct our arm movement on the mouse while our eyes track this movement on the screen. Computer mice vary in their design, number of buttons, sensitivity to movement, and degree of fine motor control required.

The cursor speed can be slowed down through the control panel, making it easier for your child to learn to control the mouse. Also, look for software programs that do not require the cursor to be in a precise position to make a selection. Some software allows for a broader area of selection, so that when the cursor gets close, it selects that item. This is known as creating "hot spots." This feature can be helpful for children who have difficulty moving to and stopping on a precise spot, but can get close. There are also some preschool computer programs that respond positively to any movement of the mouse or touch of the keyboard.

Although children may initially need hand-over-hand assistance to learn how to move the mouse and to click a selection, they often catch on quickly. "Double clicking" to open a program can be tricky and takes practice. There are mice available that have separate buttons for single clicking, double clicking, and dragging, thereby eliminating the difficulty some children have combining two movements, such as clicking and holding while dragging. Windows has a "click and lock" feature for those who have problems with clicking and dragging. In addition, you can use the control panel to change how fast the double click needs to be in order to be recognized as a double click.

There are various sizes and shapes of mice now; keep in mind that your child's hand is smaller when you are buying a mouse for your computer. The Chester mouse is a smaller mouse with a single button, designed for young children.

TASH makes switches (called Switch Click, Mini Click, and Buddy Buttons) that can be used instead of a mouse to activate programs; wireless switches are now also available (it-Switch). (See Resources.) These may be helpful for a young child with Down syndrome who would like to use simple games for learning but has difficulty with a mouse. As they grow up, many children with Down syndrome do learn how to use a regular mouse for their computer activities.

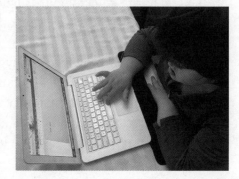

Trackpads

Trackpads are now often used with laptop computers instead of a mouse. The user moves his finger across the trackpad to direct the cursor. Using a trackpad requires the baby finger side of the hand to stabilize, while one or two fingers are used to swipe and click the trackpad. A mouse can be used with a laptop, if that is more comfortable than a trackpad.

Trackballs and Joysticks

A trackball may offer greater control than a traditional mouse, and may provide relief from the discomfort and pain that some people experience with extensive mouse use. The hand moves the ball, which in turn moves the cursor, while the rest of the unit stays in one position. Trackballs also come in a variety of shapes, sizes, sensitivities, and options. Some have speed settings (e.g., Roller Plus Trackball by Infogrip). Most trackballs have separate buttons for the click and drag functions.

A joystick is another alternative to a mouse that some children may find easier to control. The joystick is grasped with the whole hand and moved in the desired direction. As with trackballs, there are a variety of speeds, sensitivities, and sizes available.

Most computers in homes, schools, and public places are accessed using either a mouse or a touch screen. Therefore, I recommend teaching the use of a mouse, and only if there are difficulties would I recommend trying a joystick or a trackball.

Touch Screen Programs

Much of our digital interaction with the world is performed through touch screens: on ATM and bank machines, at the gas station and grocery store, at the library, and perhaps on sign-in iPads for attendance at school. The trend does seem to be moving toward touch screens and away from the use of a mouse. Touch screen options are either built into the monitor or are accessed with an external overlay that mounts on a regular monitor.

Children and adults with Down syndrome will benefit from learning how to use a touch screen as a life skill. Most will easily learn how to use a computer touch screen and touch screen tablet devices. Examples of add-on touch screens for regular computer monitors are Magic Touch from Keytec, and TouchWindow from ProEd (see Resources under Mayer-Johnson).

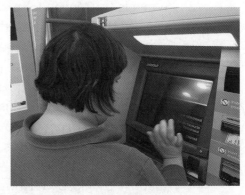
Touch screens are everywhere now.

Built-in Accessibility Options

Most computers have built in accessibility options in the control panel. For example, if you use Microsoft Windows, you can access these through "My Computer," then "Control Panel, " and then "Ease of Access Center." On Apple computers, they are found under "Applications," "Accessibility." Here are some accessibility options that may be helpful to the child with Down syndrome:

- Mouse speed: the speed that the cursor moves on the screen can be slowed down.
- "Sticky keys": two or more keys that are usually pressed simultaneously (such as shift and a letter to produce a capital letter) can instead be pressed in succession with this option.
- Keystrokes, or onscreen keyboard: rather than using the regular keyboard, the mouse is used to choose letters on the screen.
- "Filter keys" ("Slow keys" on Apple computers): the length of time a key needs to be pressed down can be adjusted. If your child unintentionally touches another key, it will not type it. The computer will type the key that is held down for the specified amount of time. Also, this option helps to avoid the problem of typing repeated letters if your child can't release the key quickly enough on the normal setting.
- Double click: double click speed can be slowed down.

Software Options

There are many software programs that help children learn keyboarding skills or develop speech and language, literacy, and other academic skills. A few of these specialized programs will be highlighted here, to give an idea of the types of programs available. See Resouces for manufacturers and distributors.

- *Picture processors:* These programs provide pictures with text. Examples are Boardmaker (by Mayer-Johnson), Writing with Symbols (by Mayer-Johnson), Kidspiration (by Inspiration software) and Clicker 6. Boardmaker is commonly used to aid many students with communication difficulties who use picture communication. The software produces representational black-and-white or color pictures depicting many common words. The pictures and words can be customized for the individual.
- *Talking word processors:* These programs provide auditory feedback for letters/words and sentences and often include word prediction. Examples are: Word Q, Clicker 6, IntelliTalk 3 (by Adaptive Synapse), Writing with Symbols (by Mayer-Johnson), and Write: OutLoud 6 (by Don Johnston), which is a simple talking word processor program without word prediction.

■ *Word prediction programs:* Word prediction programs provide word options after a few letters of the word are typed in. They can speed up writing for students who need help with spelling but can read. The software can be customized to provide options of words frequently used by that individual. Once the word is displayed, it can be chosen with a click, reducing the need for typing individual letters. An example of a word prediction program is CO:Writer by Don Johnston, Inc., which integrates with Write: Out Loud. Other examples of word prediction software are Clicker 6, Word Q, and Write Online (by Crick software, and which is aimed at higher level literacy: late primary, secondary, and college students).

Educational software options are many. For older children, teens, and adults who have Down syndrome, the challenge is to find software that is appropriate for the chronological age of the user, while still providing learning content that is appropriate for their cognitive and learning level. There is a need for appropriate levels of content and design presentation (26).

Summary of Technology Options

In summary, technological options for children and adults who have Down syndrome have exploded in the past few years. Supportive technology is more affordable and accessible with the advent of mainstream touch devices such as the iPad. Most children and adults are naturally drawn to these highly visual, intuitive devices. The focus in this chapter has been on the use of these tools to support written work, but obviously the use of computers and other devices is now an essential life skill.

Since your child will grow up to use computers in different environments (home, school, and work), it is best if he can learn to use a computer without alternate hardware and modifications. Software and accessibility options can be accessed from any computer and are easier to try on a trial basis than hardware options. Schools have some access to some specialized software and options, and most school systems hire personnel who load and set up this software.

Most children and adults with Down syndrome will not need specialized hardware to use a computer to assist with written communication, but may benefit from some of the software picture or word processing programs, such as those described above. Start with the computer resource staff in your school and school system. If you need more help, agencies and organizations that market assistive technologies can be helpful in determining what is best for your child (such as Mayer-Johnson). In some areas, augmentative communication or assistive technology clinics or institutions are also available to help you sort through the choices. There are also numerous online groups that monitor the development and applicability of new apps for persons with Down syndrome (see Resources).

Incorporating Fine Motor Goals into Your Child's Educational Program

For many children, kindergarten is their first introduction to a structured learning environment. Most children with Down syndrome, however, will have participated in some early stimulation or preschool or daycare program, where they will have had exposure to fine motor and early learning tasks. This helps to prepare them for the curriculum-based programming that they have once they start school.

Teachers take some of these factors into consideration when assessing a child's learning in a classroom setting:

1. The child's ability to express himself verbally and on paper are the primary means by which a teacher can observe a child's understanding and retention of taught material. Most children with Down syndrome have delays and difficulties with both verbal and written communication. It is important to take fine motor abilities and goals into consideration when setting up educational goals so that the child can do written work in the classroom to the best of his potential.

2. The child's ability to focus and pay attention and to initiate and complete tasks indicates his readiness and ability to learn in an academic environment.

3. The child's ability to follow routines and organize himself and his work space throughout the school day helps to indicate his overall maturity level.

The classroom is obviously a prime place for children with Down syndrome to continue to develop their fine motor skills. In the early school years, children do a lot of concept-oriented play; manipulative play for early math and spatial skills; drawing, coloring, and cutting; and beginning printing activities. As children progress through school into the higher grades, classroom activities require fine motor skills (printing, writing, drawing, and computer use), auditory skills (listening), reading skills, and verbal skills (answering questions, expressing ideas, etc.).

Most children with Down syndrome in the public school systems in North America have an individualized education program (IEP) written up, usually annually. These plans identify short- and long-term educational goals, and the strategies and resources to be used in meeting those goals. Each child's education plan will reflect his own level of development and individual needs within that particular classroom environment. In order to establish fine motor goals for the educational plan that are appropriate and realistic for your child, keep the following points in mind:

1. Know your child's fine motor developmental level. The teacher can observe the manner in which your child participates in the fine motor activities that go on in the classroom. You, as parents, can supplement this with information about what self-help skills and play activities he is able to do at home. A comprehensive fine motor assessment by an occupational therapist can give more information on the quality of fine motor movements, development of grasp and other fine motor patterns, and visual motor skills. Once the developmental level of your child's fine motor abilities is known, goals can be set.

2. Set goals in small steps. If activities are broken down into small steps and goals set one step at a time, there is a greater chance of success, everyone can see progress, and your child will probably be more motivated.

3. Reevaluate goals at set intervals. If no change or progress is seen after a set period of time, the goal should be reevaluated. Perhaps the presentation or materials need to be changed, or the goal itself changed.

4. Keep the goals relevant to your child. If he can see the point of working toward a goal and the activities used to reach that goal are of interest to him, he will be more motivated to keep at it.

Goals for Children in Classroom Settings

For children who are included in regular classroom settings, fine motor goals on their educational plan will usually reflect accommodations and modifications of the fine motor activities that the class participates in, and additions to those activities already going on in the classroom. Children who are in specialized classes all or part of the day will also have IEPs based on their individual needs and goals.

Here are some examples of goals with specific classroom activities that could be incorporated into the educational plan of a child with Down syndrome:

KINDERGARTEN—GRADE 1

Goals	Strategies
Mark will use a tripod grasp of a pencil and marker.	Pencil grip; small pieces of chalk at a blackboard; drawing at easel and at table.
Mark will demonstrate improved control of pencil movement.	Making connecting lines on matching worksheets. Circling pictures on phonics worksheets. Drawing and painting at easel. Completing preprinting worksheets.
Mark will be able to print his name.	Mark prints each letter after demonstration by EA (educational assistant). Mark prints whole name after demonstration by EA. Mark traces the letters of his name. Mark copies his name from his name card.
Mark will cut along a line with scissors.	Mark will hold scissors in the mid position (thumb on top) with help. Mark will cut two or more strokes starting close to his body and cutting out. Mark will cut along dotted lines to cut out sentence strips to match with pictures.
Mark will organize his work to take home.	Mark will roll up his paintings. Mark will fold his work papers in half and put in his backpack.
Mark will improve his fine finger dexterity.	Mark will insert his attendance card into the slot on the attendance board. Mark will put a sticker beside every activity in his activity record book upon completion. Mark will complete a 10-piece interlocking puzzle. Mark will stack and count 10 math counting blocks. Mark will unscrew the glue stick and apply glue in cutting and pasting.

Mark will unzip his lunch bag and open his juice box at lunch/snack.

Mark will use his index and third fingers to use arrow buttons for selection on the computer.

Mark will take a handful of pencils and distribute one to each child.

GRADES 2-4

Goals	*Strategies*
Katie will print independently.	Katie will practice printing the individual letters of one letter group each day to reinforce letter formation.
	Katie will print her first and last name at the top of her journal entry each day.
	Katie will copy two sentences, that she has dictated, into her daily journal, with 1/2" dark spaced lines.
	Katie will leave a finger space between each word when printing.
	Katie will check off subject areas completed by class at the blackboard.
Katie will stay in the lines when coloring.	Katie will color in her own drawings.
	Katie will pick one part of the worksheet picture to color, doing it slowly and concentrating on staying in the lines.
	Katie will color in block letters on headings of worksheets.
Katie's arm and hand strength will improve.	Katie will open and hold the school door for the class after recess.
	Katie will help erase the blackboard.
	Katie will attach her completed work papers to her activity chart using a colored clothespin.
	Katie will open and close her pencil box to take out and put away her pencils/pencil crayons.
	Katie will erase errors in printing.

Katie will improve her fine finger dexterity.	Katie will collect the library signout cards from her classmates and place them in the sign-out box.
	Katie will help distribute worksheets to the class.
	Katie will attempt to zip up her coat. After three tries she will receive help.
	Katie will count out groups of 10 popsicle sticks and put a rubber band around each in math.
	Katie will insert a tape into the tape player at the listening center.
	Katie will use individual finger movement to count out answers in math addition and subtraction.
Katie will cut out simple shapes with scissors.	Katie will cut out a large square with red dots at the corners to remind her to stop and change direction.
	Katie will cut a semicircle out of a folded piece of paper (when she opens out the fold it will be a circle)
	Katie will cut out shapes and glue to a math geometry worksheet.
Katie will be able to use a language computer program with minimal assistance.	Katie will control the cursor for selections using a trackball.
	Katie will learn the keyboard position of two new letters per week (which will be highlighted on the keyboard).

GRADES 5-8

Goals	*Strategies*
Tim will be able to do a page of legible written work in his journal and math book daily.	Tim will print and underline his name and the date at the top of his journal page.
	Tim will print on regular lined paper, double spacing the lines.
	Tim will use a ruler to draw a red line down the middle of his math workbook page to help him organize his work on the page.

He will do one math problem on each side of the red line, so that his work remains separate and easy to read.

Tim will erase errors in pencil or will use white-out for pen errors. Every second day Tim will use the computer to type his journal entry.

Tim will learn to sign his name using cursive writing.	Tim will do daily prewriting activities at the blackboard.
	Tim will practice each letter of his name individually.
	Tim will write his name on the blackboard when he has completed listed activities.
Tim's hand strength will improve.	Tim will be able to open his binder to insert papers, then close it.
	Tim will use a hole punch when necessary, to insert worksheets into his binder.
	Tim will gather up the class assignments and attach them together with a large clip or paper clip.
	Tim will thumbtack art work up onto the class bulletin board.
Tim will improve in fine finger dexterity.	Tim will open and insert pages into a Duo-tang notebook cover.
	Tim will break off pieces of masking tape and will tape art work up on the walls.
	Tim will plant individual bean seeds in a class gardening activity.
Tim will be able to pour liquids without spilling.	Tim will water the class plants.
	Tim will pour exact amounts of liquid into measuring containers for science experiments.
	Tim will pour his soup into his thermos lid at lunchtime.

Tim will be able to cut a variety of shapes and sizes with scissors.

Tim will cut out and fold three-dimensional geometric shapes (cube; pyramid; cylinder).
Tim will cut out block letters for a project heading.

HIGH SCHOOL

Goals	Strategies
Jodie will use the computer to make journal entries.	Jodie will use a word prediction program to assist her with spelling as she fills out a formatted journal entry page.
Jodie will expand her computer use.	Jodie will independently type in her name and password to access programs. Jodie will remember the location of all the letters and punctuation on the keyboard.
Jodie will practice her written signature.	Daily, Jodie and her classmates will sign the attendance list.
Jodie's dexterity will continue to improve.	Jodie will assist in the construction of hallway bulletin board displays, including tacking or stapling up photos and lettering. Jodie will collate and staple together handouts. Jodie will sharpen some drawing pencils for art class. Jodie will open her combination lock.

These goals and strategies are just a few examples of how your child can work toward fine motor skill goals in the classroom. After each goal is accomplished, refer to Chapters 8 and 9 to help you define the next goal in the developmental progress of that particular skill.

Grandma's and Grandpa's List

- Magnetized letters and numbers
- Foam letters for bathtub play
- Paint, brushes, paper
- Easel; table easels
- Large memo board
- Chalkboard, chalk
- Sidewalk chalk
- Finger crayons; egg-shaped crayons
- Crayons, pencil crayons, pencils
- Markers (various sizes and types)
- Whiteboard and erasable markers
- *Handwriting without Tears* materials
- Fun erasers (to make the inevitable erasing more fun)
- Simple coloring books with clear, simple, undetailed pictures
- Simple maze books (where the child has to follow a very simple path with his pencil)
- Simple dot-to-dot activity books
- Preschool workbooks: activity books with concepts of shape and color; same and different, etc.
- Squeeze/loop (self-opening) scissors
- Good child-sized scissors with a decent cutting blade, e.g., Fiskars
- Tweezer/tong games (e.g., Operation)
- Wikki Stix
- Magnetic drawing boards, such as Magna Doodle
- Stencils; stamps
- Construction paper
- Computer software; iPad; tablet
- Sticker books

Daily Living and Independent Living Skills

Independent Living Skills
Meal preparation;
Paid/volunteer work;
Hygiene needs;
Uses technology & machines

Daily Living Skills
Self-Help: Dressing, Eating, and Drinking; Grooming
Household Chores
Leisure Activities

Dexterity
Precise movements of hands and fingers;
Individual finger movements;
Strength of finger and thumb pincer grasp

Stability
Positions the body
and arms

**Bilateral
Coordination**
The hands work together

Sensation
Sensory awareness of body
and hand position;
Motor memory of sequences
(e.g., tying shoelaces)

Self-Help Skills

Children are very busy in their first years of life, establishing the building blocks of fine motor skills and gradually gaining the movements that will develop dexterity. Self-help skills play a special role in hand skills development:

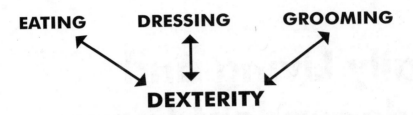

To understand the relationship between the development of dexterity and self-help skills, it may help to think about the electrical wiring that runs through a house; the current travels in both directions. It isn't necessary for a child to have developed good dexterity before she begins to do self-help activities. Practicing and doing these activities over and over will improve your child's dexterity. For example:

- Finger feeding helps to develop pincer grasp.
- Putting on socks helps to develop finger and thumb strength.
- Doing up a zipper helps to develop finger coordination, with both hands working together.

Your child will practice these tasks many, many times before they become "easy," but all that practice will develop the dexterity that she will need for other daily living skills.

Dressing

It takes years for children to become independent in dressing. Your child will gradually learn, step by step, how to undress and dress herself, fasten buttons and zippers, and make choices about her clothing. Remember the progression of learning new skills discussed in Chapter 2. Also consider these basic strategies while your child is learning dressing and undressing:

1. **Positioning:** Your child needs to be in a stable position in order to hold the clothing and put it on/off. This may mean sitting with her back against the wall to put on socks and shoes, or on a stair to push her foot into a boot.

2. **Step by Step:** As discussed in Chapter 2, a child moves gradually from being dependent to independent in dressing. Remember all the steps, let-

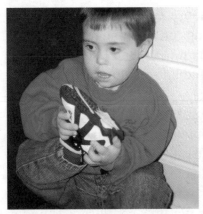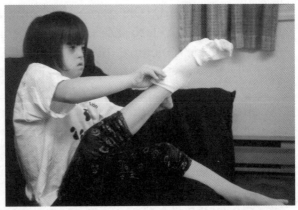

Sitting in a corner or against the wall can give a child more stability to reach down and use both hands to take off shoes or put on socks.

ting your child do more for herself as she is able. When she is beginning to learn a new skill, you can begin the task, then let your child finish the last step, or help her to finish. (This is called *backward chaining*). For example, you put the sock on over her toes, and she pulls it up over her heel. Some children respond better if you do it in the reverse order, with her starting and you finishing the task.

3. **Hand-over-Hand:** Hand-over-hand assistance works well with some children but not with others. Sarah wasn't always keen on hand-over-hand when she couldn't do things by herself; she wanted to be independent. I found that talking about our hands working together as a "team" helped her accept my physical guidance when it was necessary. Use gentle movements to help guide your child's hands. As they get older, most children need less and less physical assistance.

4. **Expectations:** Don't expect too much, but do expect your child to participate in some way.

5. **Timing:** Dressing in the morning rush may not be the best time to expect your child to attempt to learn the next step in the task. Try to find a time that isn't rushed and that is motivating, such as getting changed for swimming.

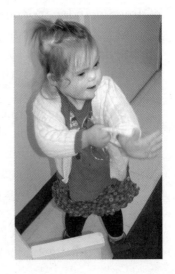

6. **Modeling:** Letting your child watch you or her siblings dress will help her through imitation. Dressing together may be more fun for her than on her own.

7. **Choice of Clothing:** Choose easy clothing: loose, comfortable fabrics, elastic waist bands, Velcro shoes. Avoid fastenings on clothing for young children when possible; e.g., use pullover shirts rather than button-up shirts and elastic-waist jeans rather than zipper- and button-closing jeans.

8. **Sequencing:** Sometimes children can manage the physical skills required in dressing but may have difficulty planning how to carry out the step-by-step sequencing required. In this case, visual cues may help. A strip of picture symbols (such as those available through the Boardmaker software program from Mayer-Johnson) showing the correct sequence for dressing can be used. For example, the pictures could say: 1. underwear; 2. T-shirt; 3. pants; 4. socks; 5. shoes; 6. sweater. If the Boardmaker program is not available, you can use pictures cut out of magazines or actual photos of your child's clothes. There are apps in which customized photos can be used to develop visual sequencing cues and visual schedules (e.g., Magnus Mode).

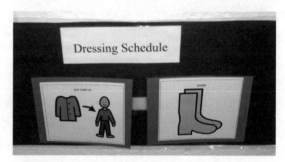

A visual schedule provides prompts to initiate and complete the steps of activities.

Usually, children learn to take off loose clothing before they learn to put it on. Babies often frustrate their parents by continually taking off their hat, mitts, or socks! If your baby doesn't do this on her own, help guide her hands to do it when you come in from outside or are getting ready for bed. This stage is important for your baby to develop a sense of body parts and the first steps of dressing independence.

As your child develops, you will gradually increase the expectations during the daily routine. Here are the main steps in dressing skills that our children learn. They are outlined in approximate order of difficulty, but your child will usually be learning several skills at once:

- Taking off hat; mittens
- Taking off socks and shoes
- Putting on hat
- Taking off jacket (after it is undone)
- Pulling down pants and taking off
- Pulling shirt on/off the head
- Pulling zippers up and down (once started)
- Putting on jacket using the flip method (described below)

- Taking off loose pajamas
- Putting legs in pants and pulling up
- Putting arms in sleeves of shirt (once over head)
- Putting shoes/boots on
- Putting socks on
- Pulling arms out of sleeves
- Putting shirt over head and putting arms through
- Putting on jacket (usual method)
- Putting on a front-opening shirt/blouse
- Buttoning
- Zipping up (including starting)
- Tying shoelaces

Common Dressing Challenges and Solutions for Children with Down Syndrome

Putting on a Jacket

The flip method is often taught to young children in day cares and nursery schools, as it may be easier for them to do than the usual method. Your child sits or stands on the floor. Lay the jacket down on the floor, with the top of the jacket label/hood closest to your child and the inside of the jacket facing up. Your child pushes her arms into the armholes and then flips the jacket up over her head.

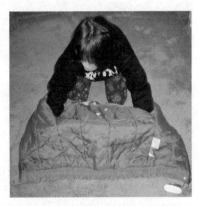

Young children can learn to put on their coats using the flip method.

Another approach is to place the hood of the jacket on your child's head. The jacket is then in position for her to put her arms into the sleeves. This technique can be a good transition between the flip method and the regular method, as your child has to reach behind to slip her arms into the sleeves when the hood is on her head.

When helping your child learn the regular method, have her hold the jacket with one hand above the arm hole of the other side. (For example, hold the jacket with her left hand above the right armhole). She then slips that arm in. That part is easy, because she can see where to put her arm. She then has to rotate her other arm in and behind her, find the hole, and slip her arm through, all without

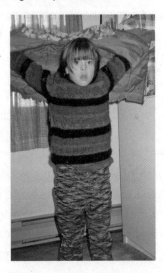

being able to see. During this step, you can help by lightly positioning the jacket so she can more easily find the sleeve behind her. Once the motor pattern becomes automatic, she will be able to find the sleeve with that arm. Most of us always put on our coat or jacket the same way, starting with the same arm. It may be easier for your child to learn if she starts with the same arm. With repeated practice, the movements become automatic.

Buttons

Fortunately, clothing for children is not encumbered with as many buttons as in years past. Elastic waist pants are popular with young children, even in blue jean styles, as are pullover sweatshirts and T-shirts. However,

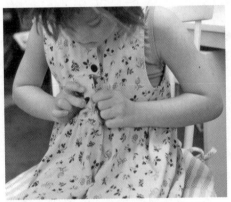

Stable positioning, a vertical buttonhole, and a clear view of the button will make buttoning easier.

as your child gets older, she probably will want to wear some styles with buttons, as her peers do. In helping Sarah learn to manage buttons, I have found that it is much easier initially to both do up and undo buttons with a vertical buttonhole, as opposed to horizontal. With a vertical buttonhole, the button just slips straight into the hole, without the wrist movement required of a horizontal buttonhole. Larger buttons and buttonholes are easier to manage than smaller buttons.

If your child is practicing on a doll or a practice button board—often found in preschool and kindergarten classrooms—it will help your child more with her own clothing if the doll or practice board is on her lap facing out. This way the buttons are facing the way they would be on her own clothing. It may be fun for your child to have "dress up" clothes with buttons, such as an old adult shirt or vest with the sleeves cut short, the buttonholes enlarged, and larger buttons sewn on.

Zippers

Children can practice zipping and unzipping on backpacks, pencil cases, etc. These provide practice and strengthening opportunities.

We all know how tricky zippers on jackets and coats can be for many children! When buying a coat or jacket for your child, look for a sturdy zipper with a stable end that is large enough to be grasped firmly. A young child will likely need help connecting the zipper to start it, then she can pull it up. Sometimes a small key ring or other attachment to the zipper tab is useful if her pincer grasp is not yet strong enough to pull up the tab. Your child may have to be shown how to hold down the base of the zipper with one hand, while pulling up the zipper with her other hand.

Trying a different position while putting on the jacket may also help. Sitting on a chair or step when connecting the zipper may be easier for your child than standing up. Here are some possible alternatives to use while your child is learning to do up zippers:

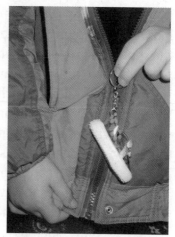

A zipper ring can make zippers easier to handle if your child has difficulty grasping the tab to pull it up and down.

1. Look for a pullover jacket with a zipper neck closure so your child can avoid the difficulty of connecting the zipper to start it.
2. Use a one-piece snowsuit.
3. Look for a coat with loop and Velcro tab closures.
4. Have your child connect the zipper with the coat on her lap and zip it up just a bit. She then steps into the coat and pulls it up and on and then completes zipping. (It is easier to connect a zipper when you don't have to bend forward and look down.)
5. Purchase a jacket with snap closures. Usually I find that snaps are more difficult than zippers, but some children may find them easier.

Shoelaces

There are many alternatives to conventional shoelaces:

- Elastic laces with easy fastening systems that allow shoes to be slipped on, such as "Lock-laces" and "Hickies"
- Shoes with Velcro closures
- Shoelace closure options, such as "Shoe-lock," "Lace Anchors," and magnetic closures

Most of these can be found in pharmacies, athletic footwear stores, or online.

Once your child is out of elementary school, you will find that most styles worn by teenagers do have standard laces, so it is a good idea for your child to learn how to tie them.

Tying shoelaces requires dexterity, the ability to sequence the movement steps involved, and enough practice that these movements become automatic. Attention, concentration, motivation, and persistence are necessary. When I wrote the first edition of this book, Sarah couldn't yet tie her shoelaces completely independently, but she did part of the process, needing help to finish. Eventually she did learn the whole sequence, and she can also double-knot them so they don't come undone. Now she is a typical young adult, tying laces loosely and slipping her feet in and out of her running shoes without touching the shoelaces. However, when necessary, she can tie them!

There are different ways to tie shoes, and you may need to experiment with your child to find out which way will work. I would *not* attempt learning to tie shoelaces if your child cannot yet do up buttons or start a zipper. It isn't necessary to know right from left. Tying shoelaces is a motor sequencing activity, and once the motor pattern is established, your child will be able to do it automatically.

1. The first step, crossing one lace over and then under the other lace, is probably the easiest part, and it is a useful thing to know how to do. Your child can practice tying on larger materials initially, such as a housecoat belt, the sash on an apron, the handles of a plastic bag, or a ribbon around a stuffed toy's neck

2. Then she can practice on a shoe that is on the table in front of her, facing out, as if it were on her foot. (Bending down to tie laces when the shoe is on the foot is more difficult for balance and stability.) When she knows how to tie the laces together, she can attempt to do so when her shoe is on!

3. After the initial tie is accomplished, the next steps can be approached in different ways:

   - Your child can either make two "bunny ears," holding one loop with each hand, which she then crosses over and under to tie together.
   - She can make one loop and hold it, while her other hand wraps the remaining lace around and tucks it under. This method is probably more difficult perceptually.

Some strategies that may help:

- Remember that wide, flat laces are easier to hold and manipulate than thin, round laces.
- Much of the difficulty with tying laces is the sequencing and the perceptual differentiation of which lace goes where. You can try using two different-colored laces, tied together at the base of the holes (you will probably have to cut them or they'll be too long). This way, your child makes one bunny ear of each color and then makes a tie with one color going over and under the other. Or, using the other method, she makes the loop with one color and wraps around and through with the other color.
- When helping your child, try to help from behind or beside her, so that your hands are oriented the same way as hers, and you are not demonstrating in reverse.

■ Backward chaining, in which an adult begins the activity and completes all but the last step, can be a helpful approach to learning to tie shoelaces. You let your child do the last step—in this case, pulling the two bows to tighten the knot. Your child learns the sequence one step at a time, beginning with the final step and proceeding backward through the sequence. With this method, the child feels the success of completing the task.

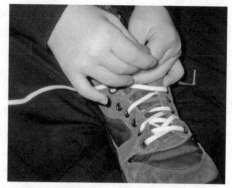

Inserting different colors of shoelaces may help the child who is learning to tie shoes.

Putting Shoes on the Right Feet

We are advised not to worry about our kids putting their shoes on the wrong feet. After all, how many thirty-year-olds do we see walking around with their shoes on the wrong feet? However, I know that many parents *would prefer* that their child learn to put shoes on the correct feet, especially if they have just paid for good orthotics for the shoes. Marking the shoes with an R or L doesn't usually work, because many kids can't consistently tell their right from left foot. I have found that putting a mark of some kind (e.g., a red dot) on the inside of each shoe at the heel works for many children. The child then puts the dots together (most children understand the concept of apart/together from about age three on), and the shoes are then lined up on the correct side.

Removing Clothes

When taking off their clothes, some children pull from the top of their sleeve or pant leg. They are usually successful at removing the article of clothing, but it is then inside out for the next time it has to be put on. It can be frustrating if every time your child has to put on her jacket, the sleeves are inside out and have to be turned for her. Teach her to grasp and pull from the bottom of the sleeve or pant leg.

Putting on Shoes

It can be difficult to put shoes on young children with Down syndrome due to low muscle tone. Their toes and forefoot might curl under as you try to slip the foot into the shoe. If you are experiencing this problem, look for shoes that have a deep enough opening with either laces or Velcro, so that it opens up right down to the toe area. You can then position the toes and forefoot more easily in the shoe. Often, children and adults have short, wide feet, requiring wide shoes. Finding shoes for Sarah that are comfortable and supportive, yet stylish, has always been a challenge for us. For day-to-day use, Sarah wears New Balance running shoes, extra wide.

Removing Shoes and Socks

I have worked in an inclusive preschool setting for almost twenty years. Inevitably, year after year, the bus drivers have one or two children who remove their shoes and socks while sitting in their car seats on the bus. And inevitably, it is always a child who has Down syndrome! We really don't know why this is, but we can speculate. Could it be that they are looking for something to do during the ride, and the shoes and socks are the only handy thing? Or could it be a sensory reason? Many young children with Down syndrome do prefer to remove their shoes and socks indoors as well.

I don't have the answer, but know that if your child does this, you are in good company! It is a stage that the child eventually outgrows.

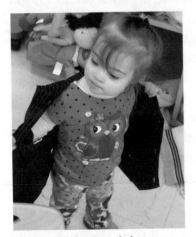

Playing with dress-up clothes provides a fun opportunity to practice dressing and undressing.

Putting Clothes on Backward

The easiest way to get around this challenge is to choose clothes that look the same whether they are on forward or backward. Track pants, T-shirts, and sweatshirts with either no pattern or with the same pattern both front and back fit this bill.

The key to getting clothes on the right way is to get started with the leg/arm going into the correct opening. I used to lay Sarah's clothes out for her to help her with this. She didn't care when things ended up on backward, so I had to decide how much I cared! (It depended on where we were going.) As she got older, she began to identify the tag as being at the back and was able to figure out the orientation of the clothes that way.

Eating and Drinking

Finger Feeding

Children with Down syndrome can begin to feed themselves with their fingers from about the age of ten to twelve months. Initially, they will hold a cracker or teething biscuit to chew on. During the next few months, they can develop the ability to pick up small pieces of food using a pincer grasp. Although a neat pincer grasp usually develops later in children with Down syndrome, do not hesitate to place small pieces of food on the highchair tray for your child once she is able to chew and swallow and does not choke on solid pieces. Babies can manage soft solid pieces (such as soft cheese and bits of banana) before they have teeth. If your baby can't pick up the pieces off the

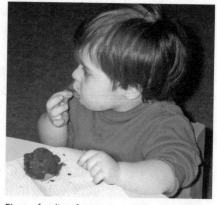

Finger feeding from a young age helps a child learn independence and self-help skills, as well as finger dexterity.

tray initially, hand her small pieces that she can grasp with her thumb and fingers and put in her mouth.

Using a Spoon and Fork

By approximately twelve to eighteen months, your child will be ready to hold a spoon. At first, just let her hold it and bang it on the highchair while you feed her. As she becomes more interested in the process, you can gently assist her in the scooping motion and in bringing the spoon to her mouth. Gradually reduce the amount of assistance you provide. Child-sized spoons with easy-to-grip handles are best to begin with. Spoons that angle inward reduce the amount of wrist movement required to get the spoon in the mouth and are easier for very young children. Examples, among many options, are the Learn 'n turn Adjustable Training Spoon and the Sassy Less Mess Angled spoon. Spoons with flat, shallow bowls are easier to eat from. It also may help initially to use the child dishes that have raised sides and suction bases, so your child can scoop against the sides. Textured foods that will stay on the spoon will be best to practice with initially, such as pudding, oatmeal, thick stews, yogurt, and pureed baby foods.

Children usually hold their spoon or fork in their palm with a palmar grasp for a few years at least, before they switch to holding it with the more mature tripod grasp that most adults use, with the thumb up. The palmar grasp may persist longer in children with Down syndrome, but when they have been

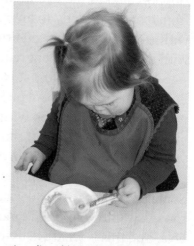

An adjustable angled spoon helps the young child orient the spoon into her mouth.

able to use a dynamic tripod grasp on a pencil for some time (see page 143), they should be able to use the more mature grasp on cutlery as well. Sometimes it is just habit that causes earlier patterns to persist. Also, the type of grasp used on cutlery has cultural and regional variations. Many adults hold their forks in a palmar grasp. If it is important to you to help your child learn to hold cutlery in the tripod grasp with her thumb up, try putting a sticker on the end of the handle of the spoon or fork. Then help her hold it so she can see the sticker.

Learning to hold and use a fork involves the same process as learning to use a spoon. Introduce using a fork with mashed or soft, chunky foods that are easy to stab and will stick to the fork, such as mashed potatoes, squash, scrambled eggs, or thick stews. Progress to soft foods that can easily be stabbed to be picked up, such as pancakes, macaroni and cheese, tender chicken, or fish. Foods that are hardest to eat with a fork are those that need a firm stab to stay on the fork, such as salad, vegetables, and meat.

As with all fine motor skills, stable positioning in a chair or high chair, with back and foot support, will help your child isolate the arm and wrist movements necessary to successfully feed herself with a spoon and fork.

Drinking

There are many cup options available when you are ready to transition your child from a bottle to cup. Drinking sets, such as the mOmma Developmental Drinking Set, include parts to transition from bottle, to sippy cup, to straw cup. Most babies go from a bottle to a non-spill sippy cup, such as the Tommy Tippee sippy cup. Some babies then transition to a straw cup, such as the Nuk. Drinking from a cup with a lid with a few small holes, such as the Hoppop, makes the eventual transition to an open cup easier. Transitioning from a bottle directly to an open cup can be difficult initially for many babies with Down syndrome, due to low tone in oral-motor muscles and difficulty with the wrist movement required to regulate the flow of liquid.

Your child may find it easier to grasp a cup with handles at first. As she develops better control of picking up and placing down the cup, you may wish to try a small child's cup without handles, to help strengthen the thumb joint and "cupping" position of the hand.

Learning to drink from a straw is a useful skill for your child to learn, in preparation for drink containers typically used at school for snacks and lunch. Some straw cups are squeezable, which enables you to squeeze the liquid up the straw into your child's mouth so she gets the idea. Juice boxes are squeezable, and this is what we used to help Sarah learn. Squeezing the cup or juice box helps the child figure out how to suck the liquid up through the straw.

Your child will gradually gain skill with cup drinking if she can practice it at every meal. Initially, your child may tip too much liquid into her mouth at once, resulting in sputtering and coughing. You can slow the liquid flow down by using nectars instead of juice, or by adding a bit of gelatin powder or infant cereal to thicken it.

It is not unusual for children to take some time to adjust to drinking from a cup when they are used to the bottle. Your child with Down syndrome may display some typical patterns:

- **Biting the Cup:** This makes for messy drinking, as the liquid can't enter the mouth if the teeth are clenched on the cup. Rest the cup on the lower lip; don't put the cup in as far as the teeth. Tell your child to "use your lips" while you gently bring her lips together on the rim of the cup.

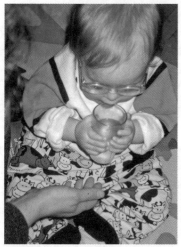

- **Protruding the Tongue:** Many young children with Down syndrome rest the cup on their tongue rather than on their lower lip when they are learning to drink from a cup. As oral-motor skills improve, they will gradually be able to keep their tongue in their mouth and use their lips on the cup. You can help your child prepare her lips for closure on the cup by tapping and stroking her lower lip to increase sensory awareness. Remind her to keep her tongue in and use her lips on the cup. At times, we used a mirror with Sarah, and she became good at self-monitoring herself while drinking.

This little boy is learning to drink from a cup.

Cutting and Spreading

Cutting and spreading with a knife are good practice opportunities for developing finger coordination and strength. The index finger guides the knife while the rest of the hand holds it stable. Complete independence in cutting of foods may not happen until your child is in late childhood or adolescence.

Often before children are given knives to cut their food, they have practiced cutting skills with play dough. Then your child can begin practicing

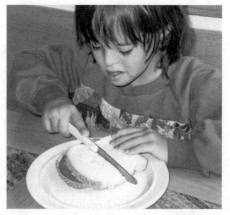

Using a knife to cut and spread helps the school-aged child develop control, which carries over to paper-and-pencil activities.

with a small, dull table knife on soft foods, such as pancakes. Encourage your school-aged child to spread her own bread or toast with butter/jam, etc., or to help you spread frosting on cupcakes. Not only will she be one step closer to making her own lunch, but this spreading practice will help her develop better control for gluing, printing, and writing at school.

As your child gets older, she will learn to cut foods such as meat. You may need to point out visual cues to help her remember which side of the knife is for cutting (the food side), and which side is for holding. There may be a serrated, bumpy, or rounded edge on the cutting side.

Oral Motor Control

It is not unusual for children with Down syndrome to experience some difficulties with oral motor control when eating and drinking. Hypotonia in the tongue, lips, and throat muscles, and a protruding lower jaw—which can make biting and chewing more difficult—can all contribute to delayed oral motor control. The following are some problems that are sometimes seen:

- difficulty coordinating suck-breathe-swallow pattern;
- choking, gagging, or aspirating (when liquid enters her airway)
- difficulty making the transition from pureed to lumpy and solid foods;
- tongue protrusion;
- poor lip closure;
- lack of complete closure of the *velum* (soft palate) during a swallow, causing some food to enter the nasal passages.

If your child has difficulty with the oral motor aspects of eating or drinking, consult with a speech-language pathologist or occupational therapist who has experience in feeding issues. Some considerations could include the following:

- positioning for feeding
- timing of feeding (e.g., allowing more time between sips or spoonfuls for swallowing)
- thickening of liquids
- graduated progression from pureed foods to solid foods
- sensory aspects of foods
- oral-motor preparation, such as tapping the muscles of the cheeks and jaw and stroking the lips

Resources related to feeding, eating, and drinking include:

- *The Down Syndrome Nutrition Handbook* by Joan E. Medlen
- *Feeding and Nutrition for the Child with Special Needs* by Marsha Dunn Klein and Tracy A. Delaney
- *Pre-Feeding Skills* by Suzanne Evans-Morris and Marsha Dunn Klein

Grooming

As with dressing and eating, children gradually develop independence in grooming and bathing over several years. Being able to care for body hygiene, teeth, hair, and toileting needs requires a combination of sensory awareness, dexterity, and social and emotional development.

Tooth Brushing

It is important that our children with Down syndrome receive consistent, daily dental hygiene at home, and regular dental care. There is a higher risk of gum disease in Down syndrome, and there can be other dental needs that require attention. Even before your baby has any teeth, you can get her used to the routine by rubbing her gums with a damp cloth or baby toothbrush. Nuk makes a toothbrush that is suitable for this purpose. By starting when your child is still an infant, she becomes accustomed to regular mouth cleaning with a brush.

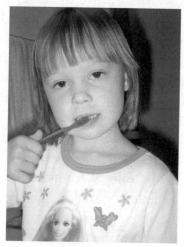

After your child brushes her teeth, an adult should go over them to make sure they are cleaned thoroughly.

Check with your dentist about the best toothbrush for your older child. An angled brush may make it easier to reach tricky spots. An electric toothbrush may be recommended for the older child and adult. Regular tooth brushing may require parental monitoring or assistance for some years, to ensure that your child is reaching all parts of her mouth and avoiding plaque buildup.

You may find that your child has decreased awareness of bits of food stuck in the mouth and difficulty removing bits with her tongue. This may mean that the food remains stuck to her teeth until they are brushed. Brushing after meals and snacks is clearly the ideal situation.

Although you may need to supervise your child's brushing, she can still participate in the routine of brushing her teeth. You can let her brush first herself and then go over her teeth again when she has finished. She can unscrew or uncap the toothpaste tube, squeeze the toothpaste onto her brush, turn the water on and off, and prepare the cup of water. These aspects of the toothbrushing routine can help develop and reinforce fine motor skills.

Pediatric dentists (specializing in dental care for children) have more appropriately sized dental chairs for children and may offer helpful distractions such as movie screens! Some health centers provide dental services, including sedation, for children and adults who are unable to tolerate dental procedures in a regular dental office.

Toilet Training

The development of bowel and bladder control is quite variable in children with Down syndrome, with many families starting the process at two to three years of age. Some children are trained within the typical period of one to two years, while others take much longer. As with typically developing children, girls seem to achieve bowel and bladder control before boys, although this isn't always the case. Begin when you feel your child has some understanding of what is expected of her, can recognize when she has had a bowel movement or has a wet diaper, can indicate her need, can sit for five minutes at a time, has a predictable bowel movement pattern, and stays dry for about two hours at a time.

Toileting is usually learned very gradually, over a long period of time. Everyone involved in your child's care (e.g., day care staff) must provide consistent toileting opportunities. I found a consistently timed toileting routine helped Sarah learn the necessary skills. She learned that she was taken to the toilet at frequent, specific times every day, and thus initially became "schedule trained." This method can work if you can recognize some predictable patterns in your child, and can use the potty with her when you know it is the right time.

Balance and stability affect a child's comfort on a toilet. Your child should have some support for her feet when sitting on the toilet and something close by to hold on to with her hands. It is usually easiest to provide a small potty for a young child, so she can help push through her feet when she is having a bowel movement. There are potties available that can be used either as a separate potty or as an insert for a regular toilet. Some have stepstools and grab handles.

If you use an insert on the regular toilet, try to choose one with grab handles and use a footstool for your child's feet. Be aware that it may be difficult for children who are on a regular-sized toilet to reach for and break off the toilet paper without feeling unbalanced. It may be easier for your child to prepare the toilet paper before sitting on the toilet. Boys can be taught to stand at the toilet to urinate.

Wiping effectively after a bowel movement can be difficult for some children and adolescents with Down syndrome. Here are some possible reasons:

- difficulty with the body and arm rotation (turning) required to reach;
- shorter arms, making it more difficult to reach;
- decreased sensory feedback (knowing when she feels clean);
- weak grasp, resulting in not enough pressure used through the hand and arm to wipe effectively.

If your child has difficulty wiping, the following suggestions may help:
- Have her stand up and hold the counter or some other surface (or grab rail) with the other hand. This will help her feel more balanced and secure for turning and reaching behind.
- Teach your child to use three (or more, as necessary for your child) separate wads of toilet paper and to wipe three times. This should be adequate to clean.
- Moist disposable wipes may be more effective for your child to use. They are also more comfortable than several wads of dry toilet paper, especially if your child has sensitive skin.
- Use of a bidet after toilet use.
- The ideal solution is a toilet used in some parts of the world that provides a cleansing spray of warm water. These are not standard issue yet in North America, but are available.

Bathing and Showering

Because independent sitting and good sitting balance develop late in children with Down syndrome, you may find it helpful to invest in some kind of bath seat for your baby or young child. Even with this support, do not assume that it is safe to leave your young child, even for a minute. *Never* leave your young child unattended in the bathtub.

The bathtub can be a fun place for you and your child to play together, while improving fine motor skills:
- scooping and pouring with various sized containers;
- dropping toys into the water (to develop release);
- using squeeze/spray bottles (hand strength);
- squeezing a puffer under water to make bubbles (hand strength);
- wringing out a washcloth (hand strength and wrist movement);
- pouring liquid soap/shampoo into your child's palm (wrist rotation, hand cupping);
- body awareness and naming body parts;
- bath mitts or puppets (sensory awareness; opening/closing movement of thumb and fingers);
- playing with foam letters/numbers that stick to the tiles when wet;
- making the shoulder movements needed to wash the opposite shoulder and the back of the neck develop shoulder mobility that will help your child when dressing herself;
- briskly drying with the towel, which gives sensory input to the muscles.

Older children and teenagers should be taught how to take a shower. It is much easier to wash your own hair in the shower than it is in the bathtub. Independence in showering will be a great asset for participation in school physical education programs, swimming, and other sports programs. If your child has difficulty with balance in the shower, you can use a nonslip bath mat, install a grab bar, or use a bath bench in the shower stall. These are available at medical supply stores. It is usually easier to squeeze some liquid soap onto a cloth or sponge than to use a bar of soap.

Hair Care

When washing your child's hair, she can practice her fine motor skills by pouring or squeezing the shampoo into her palm. Rubbing the shampoo into her hair encourages individual finger movement and sensory awareness. A small mirror suctioned on to the wall of the shower may help your child check to see if all the shampoo has been rinsed out.

Brushing hair develops wrist and shoulder movement control, especially when reaching for the back of the head. As much as possible, it is best for your child to participate in her own hair brushing. As with all of the self-care routines, try to find a pattern or rhythm to the activity that can help your child remember to complete the activity. You may want to teach her to count out a specific number of strokes for brushing each section of the hair. For example, "Brush 1, 2, 3 in the front, 1, 2, 3 in the back, 1, 2, 3 on one side, and 1, 2, 3 on the other side." Also, you can use visual cues, such as pictures of all sides of the head being brushed in sequence.

I have found that hair care can be difficult for many families, especially as children get older. If you work on these skills when your child is younger, hair brushing may go more smoothly as she gets older. Choosing an easy-to-manage hair style is sometimes necessary to make life easier, especially if your child resists brushing. Use of a softer bristle brush may be somewhat helpful. Resistance to hair brushing and haircuts may be a sensory response and is discussed in Chapter 11.

Grooming for Teens and Adults

Throughout adolescence and into adulthood, your child will continue to learn skills to manage his or her own grooming and hygiene needs. These include

- using deodorant
- shaving
- trimming and polishing nails
- menstrual care
- using facial cleansing products

- applying and removing make-up
- applying hair products and blow drying hair

Most adults with Down syndrome are able to learn how to manage these needs. As with learning all new skills, they may benefit from demonstration and modelling, breaking down the activity into smaller steps and learning one step at a time, and the opportunity to practice at routine times on a daily basis.

It is beyond the scope of this book to cover the full range of self-help skills our children need to learn and all possible strategies that can help them. What I have hoped to do is provide a framework for understanding some of the motor aspects of learning these skills, which can be improved through practice and adaptations. There are several resources for parents to turn to for detailed approaches to teaching self-help skills to children with developmental disabilities. Some are listed at the end of this chapter.

Profile: Michael

Five-year-old Michael had just started kindergarten in a regular class. It soon became apparent that he wasn't participating in the routine of coming into the classroom and removing his outerwear with the other children. When he came in, he simply stood at the door, waiting for someone to assist him. His teacher, rather than helping him immediately, attempted to determine how much he was capable of doing. When she asked him to unzip his jacket, the zipper tab slipped out of his fingers, and he quickly gave up. When she handed him his coat to hang up, she noticed that he lost some control of his balance when he lifted his arms to reach for the hook, so that he couldn't get the coat on the hook.

After a meeting with the parents, teacher, and consultant occupational therapist, a few strategies were put into place to help Michael be more independent in this routine. He was given a zipper ring, which is easier to grasp than the zipper tab, and enabled him to unzip his jacket. The coat hook was lowered and put at the end of the row so he could easily reach it, and he wasn't jostled as much by the other children. When winter came, Michael was given a low bench to sit on so he could remove his boots (slip-on style, without laces), and put on his shoes (Velcro-closure running shoes). With these adaptations, Michael soon became independent as he came into school, and he gained confidence in greeting and interacting with his classmates. By first grade he no longer needed the adaptations.

Household Tasks

As our children mature, we hope they will begin to assume the role of helper in our home. Encouraging your child to participate in household tasks from a young age has many benefits. Your child learns that every family member has a role to play in household chores and that she can make a meaningful contribution. Just don't expect a perfect job! She will not be able to make the bed as neatly as you can, but what is more important is that she will develop the confidence to do it and the positive self-esteem from having completed a task.

Many young children go through an imitative stage (at about two to four years), during which they love to imitate their parents around the house. Later, they often go through a helpful stage, in which they actually want to help and genuinely enjoy doing tasks for you. As they get older, however, you are probably more likely to face resistance to household chores!

In the chapters on stability, sensation, and bilateral coordination, several references were made to household activities. Activities such as sweeping, folding towels, vacuuming, dusting, etc., are all good ways to improve these building blocks of fine motor skills in your child. Whenever she participates in these activities with you, she is improving her stability, bilateral coordination, and sensory awareness in her hands, arms, and body. Many of these activities will also help your child develop dexterity, the fine movements of her hands and fingers.

Chores Your Child Can Participate In

Examples of appropriate household activities for a child with Down syndrome include the following:

1. **Tidying Up Toys:** You can start teaching your child to tidy up when she is very young and is learning to grasp objects and release them into containers. Putting away toys can help your child learn to identify *same/different* and to sort as she puts them into the appropriate container. Toddlers and preschoolers can practice throwing skills by tossing blocks into the bucket.

2. **Setting the Table:** Your child learns to count the correct number of utensils needed and to hold them in her hand while placing them down one at a time on the table. She learns spatial organization when making a place setting. Carrying plates is good for wrist and hand strength and wrist rotation.

3. **Assisting with Meal Preparation:** When assisting you with baking or cooking, your child can work on these skills:

  - Practice control of scooping and pouring both dry ingredients (e.g., flour, sugar), and wet ingredients (e.g., water, oil).
  - Stir and mix, which develops control and strength of grasp and wrist movements. The other hand holds the bowl steady (bilateral coordination).
  - Knead dough, which develops strength in the hands and wrists. Shaping cookie dough into balls helps the smaller movements of the fingers. Sensory awareness in the hands is enhanced when working with dough.

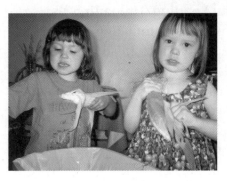

  - Vegetable preparation can include activities such as opening and removing fresh peas from the pod (bilateral thumb and finger control; pincer grasp); breaking the ends off green beans (pincer strength), or husking corn. The older child can cut soft vegetables, such as cucumbers or cooked potatoes, and can attempt to peel carrots.
  - Adolescents can help make salad by ripping and washing lettuce and cutting vegetables. They can also be involved in opening packages and cans, using measuring cups and spoons, and pouring. There are endless opportunities in the kitchen to use and develop fine motor skills!

4. **Gardening:** Children of all ages love to get their hands in the dirt in the garden! Digging helps develop strength and stability, one of the foundations for finer movements.

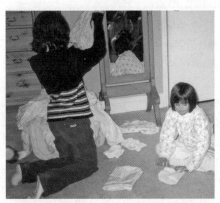

Children take pride in being able to help around the house. By participating in chores, they learn important life skills and develop their hand skills.

5. **Raking Leaves and Shoveling Snow:** Both of these activities develop upper body strength and stability and bilateral coordination. Adjusting to the weight and resistance of the snow or leaves also helps develop sensory awareness through the muscles and joints in the arms.

6. **Sorting and Folding Laundry:** Young children can learn about *same/different* by helping to sort socks. Folding flat items, such as pillowcases or towels, is a good bilateral coordination activity for young school-aged children. Folding a

towel helps your child with the control needed to bring the two sides together with a fold in the middle. This skill will help her learn to fold papers in half for putting into her backpack at school.

7. **Sweeping, Vacuuming, Washing the Floor:** Vacuuming, sweeping, and washing the floor develop body and shoulder stability, as your child moves her arms in all directions while maintaining her balance.

8. **Cleaning Windows and Mirrors; Dusting:** Spraying the window cleaner or dusting cleaner helps develop hand stability and index finger control, not to mention aim! Wiping with the cloth enhances shoulder movement and body stability.

9. **Washing and Drying Dishes and Loading/Unloading the Dishwasher:** Your child uses sensory discrimination skills to sort out dishes, silverware, etc. in the soapy water. In addition, both washing and drying are good bilateral coordination activities. And your child develops strength as she holds dishes, lifts items out of the dishwasher, and scrubs dirty pots.

10. **Putting Away Groceries:** As well as learning organizational and sorting skills, your child learns to adjust her grasp and movement to the size and shape of the item when she helps you put away the groceries.

11. **Making the Bed:** Bilateral coordination and stability are used as your child pulls up the covers and smoothes out the bed.

Leisure

Leisure activities are those we do for fun and recreation. Developing leisure interests early in life promotes a sense of well-being and an active and participatory lifestyle that will result in many enjoyable hours of free time in adulthood.

Full-time employment and family responsibilities may not fill the days of our children with Down syndrome when they are adults. Thus, it is crucial for them to begin to develop interests and pastimes that are rewarding and meaningful while they are young. These may include volunteer work, group social activities, music, dance, sports, outdoor pursuits, pets, gardening, art, theater, reading, collections, crafts, etc.

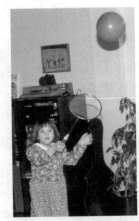

Children can get creative during play. Here my daughters have made up a "balloon badminton" game.

The list is endless! For the purposes of this book, a few possible leisure activities as they relate to your child's developing fine motor skills will be discussed.

Helping Your Child Develop Fine Motor Skills through Leisure Activities

Much of the teaching and assisting we do as parents must be structured to be successful. However, it is also important for your child to learn to initiate fun activities herself, so she can amuse herself without always needing structured entertainment. From an early age, encourage her to develop the ability to play freely, without constant adult structure. (This does not mean without adult supervision!) Below are some ideas to get you thinking about involving your child in leisure activities at home and in the community.

Community Programs: Involvement in community programs, such as Girl Guides or Scouts and Boy Scouts, youth groups in faith communities, etc., is valuable for building a sense of community and involvement, and for developing social skills in an environment outside of school.

Telephone Use: Learning how to use the telephone to call cousins, grandparents, and friends is a positive social ability that will help your child interact with peers as she gets older. Although most personal cell phones have contact numbers saved in the phone, learning to dial an unfamiliar number is good practice.

Sports and Fitness: Sports and fitness activities also offer opportunities for children and adults with Down syndrome to develop in many areas. Overall movement control may be enhanced, which helps lay a good foundation for fine motor skill development. Self-esteem, emotional development, and social interaction skills can all flourish in the right environment. Many children and adults with Down syndrome participate in community recreation programs and on sports teams. Others find the Special Olympics programs to be inspiring and rewarding. Exercise and fitness are essential components of the health of an adult with Down syndrome.

Children, teens, and adults with Down syndrome vary in their interests, just as all children do. One child may love basketball, another soccer, and another rhythmic gymnastics. Swimming and gymnastics are particularly good for developing strength and stability. Children with Down syndrome *must* be examined medically for atlanto-axial instability (with a neck x-ray) prior to participation in contact sports, skiing, and gymnastics. If atlanto-axial instability is present, it may be recommended that your child not participate in these sports, although medical opinion seems to differ on this matter. There are many sports and recreational activities that are appropriate and can be mastered by people with Down syndrome. The challenge for parents is matching the child's interests with the programs available in their community.

Over the years, Sarah has participated in many different types of sporting activities. She has now narrowed down her participation to those she likes best: swimming, dancing, walking, bike riding (a tandem bike), and baseball.

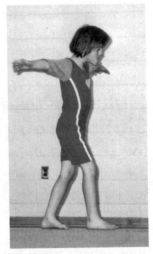

Gymnastics programs can help the child improve overall strength and endurance, which will enhance her physical well-being.

Creative and Imaginary Play: Keep supplies available for creative and imaginary play (e.g., dress-up clothes and art and craft supplies). Art and craft activities usually focus on dexterity, and require a lot of small finger movement and coordination. For this reason, children with Down syndrome may shy away from these activities. However, crafts and art can be both beneficial and rewarding for children with Down syndrome. The secret is to know your child's abilities and adapt or prepare the activity ahead of time so that she will be able to participate successfully and feel a sense of satisfaction, not frustration.

Sometimes, having the "perfect" model in front of her to try to copy is not the best idea. She will not be able to produce the same result. Creativity, and the process of doing it, is what is important.

Arts and craft activities that are openly creative and do not require a precise duplication of the model will probably be more rewarding and successful for most children with Down syndrome. Here are some examples:

- Make a frame or wreath by pasting decorative pieces of foam, sequins, etc. on to a precut shape.
- Thread decorative beads with large holes onto pipe cleaners, which can then be bent into different shapes.
- Make plaster mold kits, in which a plaster mixture, mixed with water, is poured into a plastic mold.
- Press rubber stamps on a stamp pad and then on paper; this is a good activity for strengthening the thumb and fingers in the tripod grasp.
- Make crayon rubbings by placing flat, textured items (e.g., coins, textured placemat, leaves, tiles) under a piece of paper and rubbing the side of a crayon over it.

- Create black magic pictures: Color an entire piece of paper with different colors of crayons in a random pattern. Color over top with black crayon, completely covering the other colors. Take the blunt end of scissors and scratch a drawing through the black crayon to reveal the other color underneath.
- Another way to make black magic pictures is to color a picture with crayons (fluorescent show up best) and then paint over the entire paper with black poster paint. The paint will fill in the uncolored areas of the paper, but will not stick to the crayoning, which shows through.
- Try torn tissue design: Rip pieces of tissue paper of different colors and place them around a piece of sturdy paper, overlapping the colors. Paint over all with a mixture of white glue diluted with water. This will hold the tissue paper in place and the color combinations will show up nicely. Tearing paper is a good activity for coordinating the wrist movements of both hands. Tissue paper has a grain and will only rip well in one direction.
- Experiment with fold and dye dipping: Fold a piece of absorbent paper (like a sturdy paper towel) many times to make it into a small square or triangle. Dip the corners into little bowls of food coloring. The dyes will spread and mix, giving a beautiful effect. This is a good activity to practice folding paper.
- Make a bird feeder: Attach a string at the top of a pine cone for hanging up your bird feeder. Put peanut butter all over the pine cone and then sprinkle with bird seed. Hang up outside!

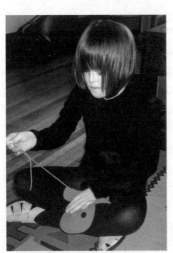

Craft activities should be simple, preferably with repetitive steps, allowing the child to improve during the activity and to feel successful.

- Create sticker art: Stick precut stickers on to a paper in a random or specific design. Peeling the sticker off the backing is good for pincer grasp.
- Make vegetable print designs: Cut fruit and vegetables in half (e.g., apple, onion, orange, cabbage), dip the cut side in a bit of paint or dye, and then stamp on a paper. Don't use too much paint or the textured effect of the vegetable will not show through.
- Make Chinese lanterns: This is a good craft activity for children who can cut straight lines. Fold a paper in half lengthwise. Starting at the fold, cut straight lines about one-half inch apart about two-thirds of the way across the paper, along the length of the fold. Open the paper and glue the sides together, then hang up.

Music and Dance: Music is another creative and leisure activity that can have many benefits for people with Down syndrome. Involvement in music programs enhances listening skills, rhythm, speech, and coordination. People with Down syndrome can benefit from music therapy as well as learn specific music skills. Learning to play an instrument develops self-discipline, finger control and speed, timing, and motor control. Listening to music, and learning how to choose and put on CDs or scroll through their iPod, is a relaxing and rewarding leisure activity for many.

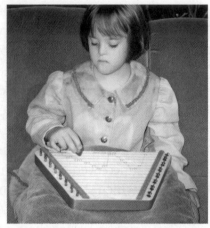

A Music Maker was Sarah's introduction to a musical instrument.

I have yet to meet a young person with Down syndrome who does not love to dance! Sarah and her friends get together once a month for DJ dances; nobody sits out even one dance! Dance is a marvelous way to achieve exercise in an enjoyable way. Like music, dancing can be enjoyed purely as a recreational activity or can be an instructional activity where the goals are remembering a dance sequence, developing timing, paying attention, etc.

Independent Living Skills

Although some people with Down syndrome live completely independently, many live in family, personal relationship, community, or group settings, like most of us. Within our living situations, we all assume various roles and responsibilities. We make decisions and carry out day-to-day tasks with our partners, family, roommates, etc. This is what we hope our children with Down syndrome will be able to do as they grow into adults with Down syndrome. Independent living skills are those that will help adults who have Down syndrome engage actively in living arrangements with friends, family etc. Some of those skills are mentioned here:

- **Household Tasks and Meal Preparation:** Many of the related fine motor skills have been discussed earlier in this chapter. Other skills include emptying trash, cleaning, using keys or keypad locks, replacing batteries, using kitchen appliances and utensils, using knives safely.

■ **Personal Care and Hygiene:** Teaching self-care skills begins in childhood and continues into adulthood. Adults may take responsibility for daily bathing or showering, shaving, menstrual care, taking medications, choosing clothing, using a washing machine and dryer, folding and putting 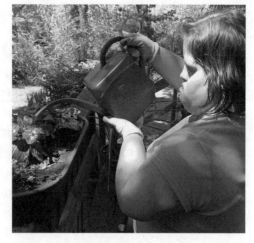 away clothes, cutting nails, getting their hair cut, choosing and doing exercise.

■ **Personal Management:** The acquisition of skills to manage and schedule their days gives adults a sense of autonomy and control over their lives. Some of these skills include using an alarm clock or phone alarm to get up on time, using a calendar to keep track of appointments and events, keeping to a regular schedule of meals and sleep, getting to and from work or programs, and organizing leisure time.

■ **Community Skills:** Skills in the community involve such things as writing checks, using an ATM machine, using a phone, using debit and credit cards, having an understanding of costs and the worth of items when shopping, safely navigating on 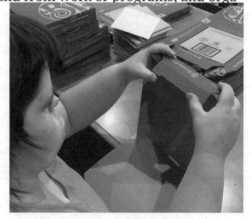 foot or by using public transportation, filling out forms, using a computer or tablet, using public services such as recreation centers and the library, and understanding personal boundaries and safety in relationships.

Many teens and young adults with Down syndrome have the opportunity to participate in employment skills training, either through education co-op programs at school or college or through community agencies. Some are able to move on to paid employment; many more would have the potential to do so if the opportunities were available.

Useful books related to teaching independent living skills include the following:

- *Steps to Independence: Teaching Everyday Skills to Children with Special Needs,* by Bruce L. Baker and Alan J. Brightman
- *Taking Care of Myself: A Hygiene, Puberty, and Personal Curriculum for Young People with Autism,* by Mary Wrobel
- *Steps to Independence Guide*, an online publication available on the website of Community Living Toronto, connectability.ca
- *Pre-Feeding Skills: A Comprehensive Resource for Mealtime Development,* by Suzanne Evans Morris and Marsha Dunn Klein (www. mealtimenotions.com)

Grandma's and Grandpa's List

- Dress-up clothes
- Old Halloween costumes
- Adapted shoelaces
- Child's kitchen and dish set; tea set
- Toys that have fastenings that promote dressing skills
- Child-sized broom and dustpan
- Child-sized shovels, rakes, and gardening set
- Doll with long hair for brushing
- Stuffed toys with ribbons for tying
- Toy lace-up boots/shoes for lacing and tying
- Nonslip bowl; adjustable, angled spoon
- Child-sized cutlery
- Graduated cups for learning to drink from a cup
- Potty seat
- Games and activities for leisure

11

Sensory Processing

In Chapter 7 I discussed sensation and how its components (touch, position, and movement) contribute to the development of fine motor skills. This chapter will go into more detail about sensory processing—that is, the integration of sensory information from all the sensory systems, and how this affects development and behavior. Motor skills are the end result of sensory processing; therefore, sensory processing contributes to fine motor and other motor skill development. Part of the foundation of self-help skills is body awareness, which develops through the sensory systems. Many other skills and aspects of your child's development are also affected by sensory processing.

This process is based on the theory of "sensory integration," which explores the potential relationships between the neural processes of receiving, registering, modulating, organizing, and integrating sensory input and the resulting adaptive behaviors (9). Some occupational therapists and researchers use the term *sensory processing* to describe the entire process, with integration being one component. *Sensory processing disorder* is now the term being used to describe difficulties in any or all levels of sensory processing.

In this chapter, I will discuss sensory processing first in general terms and then in relation to children and adolescents who have Down syndrome. My observations, discussions with other parents, and involvement in research have led me to believe that at least some people with Down syndrome have differences in how they process sensory input. This chapter may therefore be useful in helping you understand behaviors in your child that may be related to sensory processing, and may give you some strategies to help your child deal more effectively with his sensory needs.

What Is Sensory Processing?

Sensory processing is what enables us to be in a calm alert state, in order to respond in a productive manner to others and the environment. For example:

- Sensory processing is keeping a balanced posture while seated at a desk in class, writing spelling words dictated by the teacher, all the while not paying attention to the other noises around the room.
- Sensory processing is stepping aside as someone brushes against you in the hall, keeping up the conversation with your friend.
- Sensory processing is enjoying playing on the playground equipment at recess and then being able to stop and line up when the bell rings.

Sensory processing is the ongoing brain activity that allows us to choose what to focus our attention on, allows us to move efficiently, and to respond adaptively to our environment. In the words of author Carol Stock Kranowitz, author of *The Out-of-Sync Child,* we are "in sync" with what is going on around us.

We can expand the House Model to include sensory processing and other aspects of motor development.

An analogy of a home heating system may help understand how sensory processing fits into the house model. The house has a thermostat, which regulates the temperature. If the temperature goes below the setting, the heat comes on. The thermostat is like the threshold for the nervous system. At a certain level, the nerves will "fire" impulses with greater frequency and/or intensity to alert the brain to the sensory information. Below the threshold, the nervous system is still registering the information, but is not firing with the frequency or intensity needed to alert the higher brain centers to the information. Your nervous system modulates the thresholds by turning up or turning down your receptivity to different types of sensory input. Many home heating systems have a filter, which removes dirt and dust particles so they don't interfere with the efficiency of the system. Likewise,

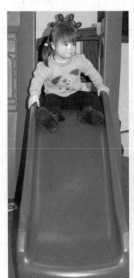
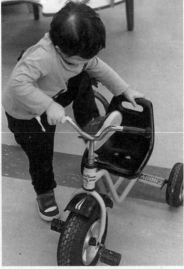

Sensory processing enables organization of responses through movement and behavior. Knowing how to use and enjoy toys such as trikes and slides are the result of sensory processing.

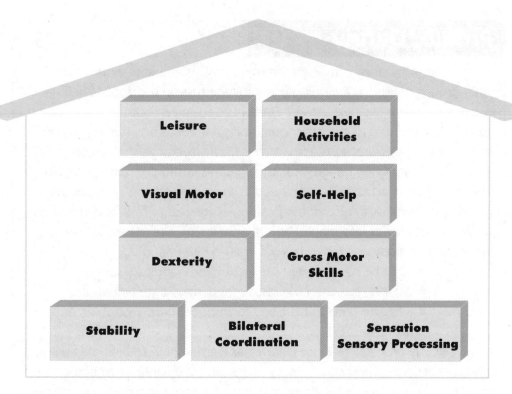

the lower areas of the brain act as a filter, screening out unimportant information so that the higher brain centers can be more *efficient*.

The home heating system regulates the temperature continuously to all levels of the house. Likewise, sensory information flows continuously to all levels of the brain, with connections between the levels and parts of the brain.

This analogy is, of course, very simplistic. The way the brain registers, modulates, interprets, and organizes sensory information is very complex, and it is also very individual. Everyone has somewhat different thresholds for sensory information, which vary according to the situation and our internal state (how tired or hungry we are, etc.). Sound is a sensory experience that clearly illustrates the concept of variable thresholds. When I am feeling "just right," high-pitched sounds (such as a baby crying) or monotonous sounds (such as a tap dripping) do not bother me. However, if I have had a long, busy, stressful day and need to concentrate on completing more tasks before I can rest, a baby crying or a tap dripping may drive me crazy. My threshold for sound has been lowered, so I am getting more information about these sounds than I need, but my nervous system is not efficiently screening them out as it normally does.

Having a "low threshold" means that it doesn't take much sensory stimulation for the nervous system to fire and to pass the information on to the conscious levels of the brain. Having a "high threshold" means that it takes a lot of sensory stimulation for the nerves to fire and pass the information along to conscious awareness.

Profile: Danny

Six-year-old Danny is taking swimming lessons at a time when several other groups of lessons are going on simultaneously in the pool. When his instructor explains the next activity, Danny has to screen out the voices of the other instructors and all the other pool noise and focus on listening to and understanding the directions. He watches his instructor as she demonstrates the starfish float. When he attempts the float, his vestibular sense gives him feedback about the position of his head in the water, and his proprioceptive system gives him awareness of the position of the rest of his body. The tactile system (touch) sends information about what it feels like to have the water supporting his body and face. Danny's brain is integrating:

- what he has **heard** in the instructions (auditory sense);
- what he has **seen** the instructor demonstrate (visual sense);
- what he **feels** in his body (proprioception, vestibular, and tactile senses).

This is sensory processing. Once Danny has learned how to float, this skill will gradually become automatic. Sensory processing will continue to occur, but he will not have to focus his attention on the sensory experience. He will be able to build upon his ability to float to learn a new swimming stroke.

Nervous System Development in Down Syndrome

As your baby grows, his brain also grows and changes. Of significant importance to brain development is the process of *myelination*. Myelin is a sheath that forms around nerves in the central nervous system and facilitates the quick and efficient transmission of information. This process of myelination is typically complete by two years of age. Research has shown that the process is delayed in infants with Down syndrome (81).

As the child grows and develops, established nerve networks are readily accessed as the foundation for new learning. New nerve growth continues as the result of ongoing sensory experiences, integration in the brain, and the connection of information in new ways. New nerve growth expands the capacity of the brain for learning and thinking. Children demonstrate their new learning in all aspects of development: movement, speech and language, cognitive, social and emotional behavior. Our unique, individual genetic makeup guides our responses to the world around us, and it is through our responses that we interact with others, learn, and develop ideas.

Nervous system development may occur more slowly in children with Down syndrome. Repetition is vital for learning for everyone; more repetition over a longer period of time is usually needed for the child with Down syndrome.

Behavior can be influenced by a number of factors. It is important to consider which factors may be triggering and reinforcing your child's behavior. Here are some questions to ask yourself:

- Is a medical condition causing the behavior? For example, a skin condition can cause discomfort and overreaction to touch; ear pain due to an ear infection may cause increased sensitivity to sound.
- Does he have difficulties with one of the senses related to the behavior? For example, does fluctuating hearing cause inconsistent attention and responsiveness to verbal instructions in the classroom?
- Is the behavior considered to be within the range of typical for your child's developmental age? For example, a three-year-old child with a developmental age of eight months who puts everything in his mouth is exhibiting typical behavior for his developmental age.
- Is the child using the behavior to communicate? For example, perhaps he wants to have a turn to be first in line going out for recess, but because he is slower getting his coat on, he is always near the end of the line. He tells you this by balking and refusing to put his coat on to go outside.
- Is the behavior a learned response (such as an avoidance technique)? For example, does he repeatedly drop his pencil on the floor to avoid doing written work?
- Is the behavior a reaction to stress that the child is unable to respond to in a more adaptive way?
- Is the behavior meeting a sensory need of the child? If you take away the behavior through behavior modification, does the child replace it with another behavior that also may be meeting the sensory need? For example, if you teach your child not to chew on his fingers, does he chew on his shirt?

As you can see from this list, there are *many* possible explanations for challenging behaviors. It often takes work and the help of professionals to sort it out and reach solutions that work for our children.

Medical Considerations

There are several possible medical reasons for some of the behaviors that will be described in this chapter. For example, lethargy and low energy may be due to thyroid dysfunction, dehydration, or sleep apnea, rather than to sensory processing. Some medical journal articles report an incidence of sleep apnea as high as 45 percent in individuals with Down syndrome. Some adolescents and adults with Down syndrome experience lethargy and low energy related to depression.

Teeth grinding (*bruxism*) is another behavior that could be due both to sensory processing or to medical issues. For example, sinus pain, tooth decay, jaw instability, and ear infection could all lead to teeth grinding. Similarly, tracheoesophogeal fistula may cause discomfort swallowing certain foods, which could be misinterpreted as picky eating or oversensitivity to food textures.

All children, teens, and adults with Down syndrome should have their medical status regularly monitored using the Health Care Guidelines published by the Down Syndrome Medical Interest Group (*Down Syndrome Quarterly*, Vol. 4, No 3, Sept. 1999). These are available online at http://www.ds-health.com/health99.htm.

Sensory Impairment

Some of the sensory input going into the brain may be somewhat different for children with Down syndrome. Therefore, the child's ability to respond may also be somewhat different. The chart below describes some of the differences that may be present in sensations going in and describes how these differences may affect the child's ability to respond. Again, some of these differences may result in behaviors similar to those caused by sensory processing disorders.

Sense Alteration or Impairment	Impact on the Child
Hearing: 1. Fluctuating hearing loss due to fluid buildup in the inner ear (caused by inflammation or infection); called conductive hearing loss	1. When fluid is present, the child will hear muffled or distorted sounds, making it difficult to interpret all that is said to him. Inconsistent responses to verbal requests and ability to follow instructions. Sometimes inattention to noises; sometimes oversensitivity to them
2. Permanent hearing loss	2. Child may need hearing aids. Some sound may be distorted and sound perception altered.
3. Research has shown that speech that is heard is processed more often in the right hemisphere, which is the opposite of most people (81).	3. May possibly be more difficult to listen and respond verbally (left hemisphere motor function) because input and response areas are on different sides of brain.

Vision: 1. Near- and farsightedness	1. Can be corrected with glasses; therefore little or no impact on the child's ability to see. May affect the child's level of caution in trying new activities.
2. Nystagmus (continuous rapid movement of the eyes from side to side)	2. May cause blurry vision and difficulty focusing. Difficulty with visual tracking. Children may outgrow this condition.
3. Difficulties with depth perception	3. May have difficulty navigating stairs, escalators, and uneven surfaces. May have difficulty jumping down, such as into a pool.
Proprioception: *(Awareness of position and movement that comes from nerves in the joints, muscles, and tendons)* 1. Research suggests that low muscle tone leads to altered proprioceptive input because of the greater degree of stretch on the muscles and tendons (33).	1. More difficult to use the exact amount of muscle force and adjustments necessary for precise and sustained movements. Greater need to watch hands while doing activities; to watch feet on stairs.
Touch: 1. Nerve conduction tests have shown that touch perception is transmitted more slowly in people with Down syndrome.	1. Slower reaction to touch information. May have difficulty making fine adjustments in hands to accommodate a variety of objects.
2. Delayed and often decreased reaction to pain and difficulty pinpointing where the pain is (15).	2. Delayed reaction to getting hurt.
Vestibular: *(The sense located in the inner ear that responds to head position, tells us about the speed and direction of movement, and contributes to the development of balance skills. It is strongly connected to the visual system)* 1. Some research suggests diminished vestibular reflexes in people with Down syndrome.	1. Balance can be delayed (more than developmental age expectations) in adolescents with Down syndrome (39). This is likely due to a combination of factors, including low muscle tone.

Developmental Delay

As mentioned above, the nervous system matures more slowly in children with Down syndrome. This is *not* a problem of sensory processing—it is a developmental delay. It is important to remember that **the primary deficit of children with Down syndrome is a genetic disorder causing developmental delay affecting cognitive, motor, language, and social development.** *There may be a sensory processing component, but sensory processing is not the root cause of all the child's delays and challenges.*

During the process of maturation, a child may develop learned patterns of behavior that persist over extended periods of time. Sometimes these learned patterns are associated initially with sensory experiences or with other factors, such as stranger anxiety. In response to a sensory experience or situation, the child establishes a behavior pattern. For example, a baby may dislike being placed lying down on a changing table. He may become fearful and quite distressed. This could be due to difficulties processing the vestibular and visual information about where he is in space, or because he doesn't like the feel of cold baby wipes on his skin. This behavior may continue as he gets older, in related situations such as lying on a doctor's examining table. He may not be experiencing the same sensory experience now that he is older, but he has learned to associate being placed lying down on a high table with a fearful response. In other words, some behaviors may originally have a basis in a sensory processing delay or deficit, but they persist as learned behavioral responses (86).

With a developmental disability such as Down syndrome, the nervous system likely has less flexibility to adapt to changing situations and new demands. Expecting the child to be able to frequently adapt to changing situations and new demands will result in a lot of *stress*. Physiologically, chronic stress changes the chemical situation in the nervous system, thereby making the nervous system even less able to respond and adapt (30). When under stress, we are all less able to learn and retain learning, and it is the same for children with Down syndrome.

It is also important for us to remember that it takes more energy for our children to meet the normal demands of a day. Obviously, when more energy is required, a child will get tired more quickly.

As a parent, I know how much we want our children to be integrated into school classrooms and community activities as their siblings and school peers are. But it is also important for them to receive specialized services, such as speech and language, physical, and occupational therapy, at various stages of their life. In addition, there may be other programs available to our children that we feel we must take advantage of so that our children can "reach their potential." All this can mean a very full plate for our children, with activities scheduled throughout the week, all demanding energy and focus.

As parents and educators, we have to be aware that constantly trying to keep up, cooperate, and comply with the expectations in all these activities over the childhood and adolescent years may lead to a buildup of stress. Yet, we certainly don't want to deny our children these opportunities. I find it is a real dilemma. When Sarah was a child and teen, I tried to be very aware of her responses as my gauge for how well she was able to handle everything. Her behavioral and emotional responses were what I had to go on, as she couldn't clearly articulate her feelings about things.

Now that Sarah is an adult, she has more choice about the environments, activities, and people she chooses to spend her time with. She also has more free time, an important part of her days. Her level of stress has decreased, she almost never has "meltdowns" anymore, and she is engaged fully in life activities that she enjoys. At times, when she perceives that her schedule is getting too busy, she clearly articulates that it is "too much." We can then discuss options for decreasing the demands that she perceives.

Stress and Behavior

Stress triggers responses in our autonomic nervous system. Think of a time when you have had to speak or perform in front of a group of strangers. You may have felt butterflies in your stomach, your heart racing, your breathing becoming faster and shallower, and your hands shaking, and you may have started sweating. You may have appeared calm and collected to others, but you were probably feeling some or all of these things inside.

Physical and emotional stress can both trigger an immediate "fright, fight, or flight" response in the autonomic nervous system, with some of these physical signs:

- pupil dilation (not due to visual impairment or lighting conditions),
- shallow, quick breathing,
- fast heart rate, increased blood pressure,
- muscle tension,
- sweating.

Extended stress over long periods of time can cause more chronic behavioral and health issues, including physical ailments (e.g., stomach aches), and mental health concerns. Stress and anxiety can reduce the chemical receptiveness of the brain to memory.

Sensory Processing

Chapter 7 discussed the development of the sense of touch and proprioception in your child's hands, as well as how these abilities contribute to fine motor skill development. Touch sensation is only one part of sensory processing. Sensory processing includes all the senses:

1. vision
2. hearing
3. taste
4. smell
5. touch
6. proprioception (awareness of position and movement provided by nerves in joints, muscles, and tendons)
7. vestibular system (awareness of head and body position in space and movement provided by nerves in the inner ear; important for balance)

Sensory Processing in Children with Down Syndrome

When Sarah was a child, she had relatively few sensory processing concerns. She had trouble with transitions and was considered "stubborn" by some of her teachers, and she went through stages where she would pick at the skin of her thumb with her fingernail. As she entered and went through her teen years, she seemed to develop more sensitivity ("overresponsivity") to some sensory input, and this has continued into her adult years. The sight of certain things causes her to gag, such as anyone wearing face paint or intense face make-up. She quickly reaches her threshold for noise in environments where several people are talking at once. At times she can't tolerate others touching her or attempting to physically guide her. Her ability to modulate her responses to these situations, which are stressful for her, depends on many factors. Sometimes she can manage to override her sensory reaction, and other times she succumbs. Over the past ten years, she has become better at recognizing potentially sensory-stressful situations and either avoiding them or incorporating her own strategies in an attempt to control her responses.

The chart below describes examples of typical behavior for many children with Down syndrome, in contrast with behaviors that are more indicative of sensory processing difficulties.

Typical Behavior vs. Possible Sensory Processing Difficulty

Typical behavior for many children with Down syndrome	Behavior that may indicate sensory processing difficulties
Displays clothing preferences and wants to make his own decisions about clothes	Is extremely picky about clothing, wearing only specific types of clothing, tugs at clothing, etc., seems overly irritated by different materials, tags, etc.
Approaches new gross motor activities cautiously; sticks to familiar activities; doesn't take motor risks	Becomes distressed or is extremely fearful of movement; resists many playground activities
Dislikes self-care routines (e.g., hair brushing, nail trimming, etc.)	Consistently resists self-care routines; may become distressed and pull away or hit out
Seems unaware of danger; misses clues in the environment to danger (e.g., doesn't notice the curb and trips over it)	Seeks dangerous situations (e.g., always climbing up on tables and jumping down); seems unaware of danger; may not react to pain
Likes strong flavors, salty foods	Will only eat a limited selection of foods; extremely picky about texture, consistency, flavor, etc.
Likes to be barefoot	Either has to be barefoot (can't stand socks or shoes) or hates being barefoot
Has to watch his hands closely while doing coordinated skills, such as doing up a zipper, tying shoelaces, or using a keyboard	Has to watch hands closely during all activities, even those that have been learned for a long time (such as scooping food onto spoon or fork); always seems awkward with hands
Tires easily in physical activity (e.g., can't run for as long as typical peers)	Seems unable to get up enough energy to initiate or complete activities
Has trouble with transitions	Is very rigid in the routines and the way things have to be done (e.g., food has to be presented a certain way); becomes very distressed over any changes in routine or environment
Needs his name called and instructions given more than once; benefits from visual cues	Can't tolerate background noise and is distracted by it; or needs repeated physical prompts to initiate when given instructions; unresponsive without excessive prompting

Sensory Modulation

One part of sensory processing is sensory modulation, which enables us to pay attention to what is important at any given time. It helps us to screen out background noises and other sensory information that is not important for the situation right now. It also brings to our attention sensory input that is important. Modulation controls how intensely we notice any particular sensory input, "turning up" or "turning down" the information as necessary (86).

A person with sensory modulation difficulties may over- or underrespond to ordinary sensory experiences. This person is either too sensitive or not sensitive enough to one or more types of sensory input. For example, a child in the classroom may turn his head to every background sound and is irritated by the feel of his socks, causing him to scratch and fidget. This sensory input is not being modulated to allow him to pay full attention to the teacher.

Our brain modulates much of the sensory information around us, which allows us to focus our attention on what is important. Otherwise, we would feel bombarded and exhausted by the constant information. The nervous system "habituates" to a lot of the stimulation around us, which means that we don't always pay attention to all the information coming from every sense. For example, because we hear the hum of the fridge every day, we don't notice it anymore. Or we may not be able to recall the color of something we see every day. Some people with neurological disorders do not filter the sensory stimulation coming in very well, and it is very difficult for them to focus attention on a task when other information is constantly demanding a response.

Overresponsiveness

A child who is **overresponsive** will show some of these signs:
- significant sensitivity to clothing,
- significant distress over self-care routines,
- an inability to wear socks or long sleeves,
- an inability to tolerate background noise,
- distress and fear with movement,
- an aggressive response to light touch; can't stand being in a crowd or lining up,
- extreme pickiness about food, tolerating a very limited number of foods,
- intolerance of changes in routine or environment.

For these children with a *lower threshold*, a small amount of sensory information causes their nervous system to overreact, placing them in an increased level of alertness. The brain perceives normal amounts and intensities of sensory input as uncomfortable initially, and if they persist, as threatening and stressful. Children who are in this heightened level of alertness all the time are on edge, and because the focus of the brain is on survival and protection, they have difficulty learning new skills.

Overresponsiveness can result in *sensory defensiveness*. In order to protect himself from what is perceived as harmful sensory experiences, the child develops defensive behaviors, such as those listed above.

Underresponsiveness

A child who is **underresponsive** will exhibit behaviors such as the following:

- seeming very slow, lethargic, and unmotivated,
- being difficult to engage in interaction; unresponsive,
- lack of awareness of changes in the environment, people coming and going, etc.

When a child is underresponsive, it means it takes more of that sensory information to make his nervous system fire in order for him to respond. He has a *higher threshold*. He may not notice when someone calls his name or enters a room, when everyone around him gets up to go for lunch, when his face is dirty, or when his clothes are all twisted on his body. He may not notice because his nervous system is not passing along that information, or it is not being registered or interpreted in a way that allows him to respond.

Sensory Seekers

A child who **seeks sensory stimulation** will exhibit behaviors such as these:

- taking unsafe risks in movement activities,
- purposefully crashing into things,
- spinning himself around for a long time without seeming to get dizzy,
- always moving; unable to be still,
- touching people and things excessively,
- excessive chewing on toys, hands, or clothing,
- constantly making a sound.

The behaviors listed for sensory seekers are often typical of very young children. One-, two-, and three-year-old children often lack the ability to delay their own impulses, are unable to attend for very long, seem to constantly be on the go, and seem uncoordinated as they develop new motor skills. Thus, it is always important to consider the developmental and cognitive age of the child before interpreting behaviors as sensory processing issues.

When a child is a sensory seeker, he craves and seeks out sensory input beyond normal expectations for his developmental age. Often these children are underresponsive and are seeking the amount of sensory input they need to meet the higher threshold needs of their nervous system. However, sometimes these children are actually overresponsive to sensory input, but instead of avoiding it, they seek one kind of input in excess to "drown out" the overstimulating and uncomfortable effects of all the other input. For example, a child may constantly hum to drown out other sounds if he is overresponsive and hypersensitive to sound. Or, he may crash into walls and furniture to override his hypersensitivity to light touch.

Combinations of Sensory Processing Problems

Often children do not fall neatly into one category, and may show components of all three sensory modulation difficulties. This is because a nervous system that is "out of sync" is going to swing more in its responses to sensory input (73).

From my experiences and those of other parents who responded to a sensory questionnaire aimed at children aged three to ten years, it seems that *some* children with Down syndrome do exhibit sensory modulation difficulties. Children with Down syndrome, as reported by their parents in this study, more often exhibit behaviors related to underresponsive and sensory-seeking sensory-modulation differences. Oversensitivity to touch related to grooming activities seems to be common, but not to other

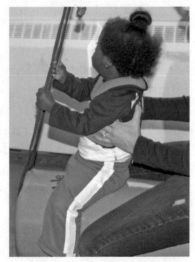

This child is wearing a pressure vest, and is swinging rhythmically forward and back on a bolster swing to help him become calm and organized for the next activity.

aspects of touch processing. Auditory processing and physical strength and stamina were also areas of concern among the parents surveyed, which is to be expected given that ear and hearing challenges and hypotonia are common. (9)

Strategies for Coping with Sensory Processing Difficulties

The following chart provides an overview of sensory processing difficulties that sometimes seem to occur in children with Down syndrome, and strategies to help your child cope. See the following table for photos of toys and equipment that can be helpful in implementing these strategies.

Examples of Sensory Processing Difficulties	Examples of Strategies to Cope
Overresponsiveness to Light Touch 1. Child is overresponsive to light touch. He may withdraw from being close to others, or may hit out if he feels threatened.	1. Approach your child from the front so he can see you and can anticipate your approach and touch. Check out the lining up, cloakroom, and seating arrangements in the classroom. Your child may be less anxious about unexpected touch if he is at the front of the line (perhaps holding the door, which provides pressure through the arms), or at the back of the line, where he can see everyone else. He may have less difficulty if his coat hook is at the end of the row or if he can go a minute ahead of the other children to put on his coat. He will feel more comfortable if no one sits right behind him. ■ Proprioception activities (heavy work through the muscles) are calming and organizing and reduce the impact of light touch on the nervous system. Examples of such activities include pushing and pulling a wagon, cart, or heavy doors; carrying heavy items; and most jungle gym activities. ■ Deep pressure touch also overrides the feeling of light touch. Tight clothing, massage, joint compressions, lying under a heavy blanket, using a weighted lap board or neck wrap, and wearing a weighted vest are examples of deep pressure touch. ■ The Wilbargar Protocol (p. 240) can help modulate the effects of light touch (75).
2. Child is extremely particular about clothing; some children don't tolerate long sleeves or socks.	2. Constant pressure input from tight Lycra clothing helps some children who are hypersensitive to the touch of clothing (e.g., exercise or bike shorts and a lycra tank top under other clothing). Certain materials are more comfortable against the skin (e.g., soft cotton, fleece). The suggestions above for touch sensitivity may also help.

3. Child avoids, resists, or fights self-care routines, such as teeth brushing, hair washing, face washing, cutting nails.	3. Encourage your child to do as much self-care himself as possible even if he doesn't do a great job. The sensory input is much more tolerable when you do it yourself, as you can anticipate the pressure and location.
	■ If this is not fully possible, do self-care routines in a consistent manner, at same place and time each day—included in visual schedule, if child uses one.
	■ Reduce impact of light touch through deep pressure, e.g.:
	  ● child hugs a large stuffed toy while hair is being brushed;
	  ● child is wrapped in a "comfort blanket" while face is washed, having hair brushed, etc.;
	  ● child squeezes a ball or pulls a thick band during self-care;
	  ● child wears exercise weights on his wrists and ankles.
	■ Cut nails while your child is in a warm bath. The warm water softens the nails, and diminishes the impact of light touch.
	■ If cutting hair is difficult, try:
	  ● holding your child on your lap;
	  ● having child sit on a low chair with his feet firmly on the floor;
	  ● brushing or combing out tangles yourself before starting;
	  ● washing hair at home just before the appointment;
	  ● using the deep pressure touch suggestions listed above;
	  ● providing your child with a visual schedule of the steps involved; including when each step is finished;
	  ● using a Social Story to frame the experience in positive language (see Resources);
	  ● providing a visual distraction (such as showing a video during the haircut). Hair salons that cater to children are more likely to offer this option.

4. Child is unwilling to hold objects in his hand, using a very light fingertip grasp, although he may hold on to one preferred object	4. Introduce new toys/objects in situations where child feels safe and calm (e.g., when wrapped in a favorite blanket; when in the bathtub, etc.). ■ Massage his hands using deep pressure to diminish his hypersensitivity. ■ Offer toys that vibrate. ■ Encourage child to weight bear through his hands and push heavy objects with his hands
Overresponsiveness to Food 1. Child is extremely picky about food; tolerates a very narrow range of textures and types of food.	1. Remember that many younger children have limited food preferences for a few years; picky eating doesn't always indicate a sensory problem. If oversensitivity is severely limiting child's nutrition, consider: ■ defocusing attention on food; try to make mealtimes important for social value; ■ including child in preparation of food (touching food, opening packages, etc.); ■ letting child touch and smell new food without any expectation of tasting it initially; ■ beginning with what your child will tolerate and gradually adjusting texture/flavor and presentation; ■ doing oral-motor activities outside of eating times to desensitize the mouth (blowing whistles and bubbles in front of a mirror, blowing bubbles through a straw, playing body parts games such as "Head and Shoulders");
General Overresponsiveness 1. Child seems to be easily overstimulated by the environment. Too much of any type of sensory input for him to process is disorganizing, and he seems unable to cope behaviorally and emotionally. 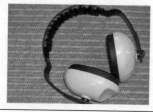	1. Change the environment by reducing the stimulation: ■ Declutter a busy room full of toys. ■ Put away toys/activities not in use. ■ Muffle sound by putting tennis balls or felt pads on chair legs, placing area rugs down, hanging banners, etc., on the walls. ■ Have the child wear sound reducing headphones in noisy environments.

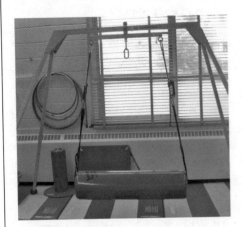

Use calming and organizing activities:
- a quiet room without intense lighting
- soft, soothing music
- rhythmic rocking, such as in a rocking chair, swing, or hammock
- warm water (such as a warm bath, or playing in warm water)
- hugs; cuddling with a pillow and stuffed animals
- chewing activities (gum, chewy food)
- provide a "quiet space," such as a corner full of pillows or a small tent where the child can retreat and reorganize himself if he feels overwhelmed
- visit a Snoezelen room (described on page 248)

2. Difficulty with sleep routines; may have difficulty falling and staying asleep; dislikes blankets.

2. Establish a bedtime routine that includes techniques such as:
- quiet activity leading up to bedtime
- cuddles; deep pressure massage
- a bath
- reading a book with a bedtime theme in bed or a rocking chair
- low lighting
- singing a lullaby

Try wearing warm pajamas with feet so a blanket may not be needed.

Underresponsiveness

1. Child needs more sensory input to be able to respond. He may seem lethargic and slow to respond. He may need more movement and sensory input before doing a focused activity to bring his nervous system up to where he can be more responsive.

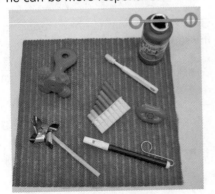

1. Prior to beginning a cognitive or motor task, try these suggestions:
- oral-motor activities: blowing bubbles or blowing through a straw; eating Popsicles or a snow cone; sucking on something sour; eating crunchy food such as carrot sticks or an apple
- quick movement activities
- brisk walking, running, jumping, bouncing
- lively singing; listening and clapping to lively music; dancing
- feeling textured toys or materials (such as Kooshballs, rubber toys, texture books, etc.) (Do not give your child anything he could bite off if he is still mouthing toys)
- cold water on face and hands

Sensory Seeking

1. Child seeks deep pressure by seeking frequent hugs, crashing into furniture, crawling in tight spaces, etc. Deep pressure can override the nervous system effects of hypersensitivity to light touch. Many children with Down syndrome seek frequent hugs; this doesn't always reflect a sensory need, but may be a learned social behavior.

2. Child may seek excessive movement, such as swings and spinning tires. He may have difficulty sitting still because his body craves movement.

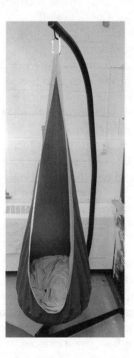

1. 2. These children need regular opportunities for movement and sensory play in a structured, predictable part of their day.
   ■ Provide structured times for the child to engage in sensory activities, trying to meet the same sensory need as those activities he craves.
   ■ Repetitive activities that provide a lot of proprioceptive input are most calming and organizing. See examples under "Overresponsiveness to Light Touch."
   ■ Other gross motor activities to try:
     ● doing modified push-ups (on hands and knees)
     ● wheelbarrow walks (holding at knees)
     ● repetitive pushing, such as a swing
     ● tug-of-war
     ● carrying heavy items, such as a stack of books
     ● jumping

(Take care not to place excessive strain on the joints. If your child is not able to hold his joints steady or if joints hyperextend beyond normal range, do not have child perform these activities.)

   ■ Household activities that provide proprioceptive input:
     ● moving laundry from the washer to the dryer
     ● carrying a full laundry basket or recycling bin (for an older child)
     ● pushing a shopping cart at the grocery store
     ● vacuuming, sweeping, and shoveling
     ● carrying a tray with heavy items on it
   ■ Provide sensory play and sensory discrimination activities for the hands.
   ■ Offer oral-motor activities at certain times during the day (such as blowing whistles, chewing gum).

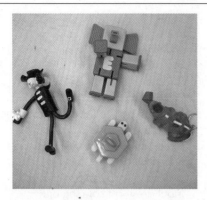

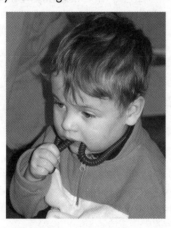

3. Child puts everything in his mouth; chews excessively on objects, shirt, etc.; may lick things.

■ Provide opportunities for some movement during circle time at preschool/school, such as sitting on a rocker board, or an inflated cushion, putting feet on a rocker board or cushion.
■ Allow the child to hold and play with a fidget toy or resistive elastic (such as Theraband) during listening times. (A fidget toys is a small toy the child can squeeze, pull, roll around in his hand, etc.).

■ Provide a "chewy" toy (can be attached to clothing using a soother clip, or use a chewy necklace or bracelet).
■ Provide other chewy toys with various textures.
■ Provide foods that are not bland, that have flavor and texture.
■ Offer thick liquids, such as nectars and milkshakes, preferably through a straw.
■ Massage your child's face, cheeks, and lips with deep pressure.
■ Offer older children chewing gum.
■ Visit dentist regularly for hygiene and to ensure that this behavior is not due to dental problems.

Motor Planning Difficulties

1. Child has difficulty learning any new motor skill, needing more practice than expected for a child with Down syndrome. A skill that he does know can't be generalized to a new situation. These children seem very disorganized in their approach to motor activities; they don't seem to know how to start and use a haphazard approach to getting through the task.

   Note that cognitive skills clearly contribute to a child's ability to quickly learn motor skills. It is still unclear how significant the sensory processing component is to motor learning in children with Down syndrome. Many children with Down syndrome do seem more dependent on environmental factors for success, however.

1. Play that incorporates a lot of tactile experiences (see Chapter 7) can be beneficial for disorganized children. Body awareness activities such as "Simon Says" or obstacle courses can help them become more aware of body position and movement.

   Having child verbalize what he needs to do to complete a task can help. For example, saying "1, 2, 3, throw" helps to focus the attention on the movement of throwing a ball accurately. Help your child develop verbal strategies and cues to complete a task. Young children often use such verbal cues when learning to print.

   Structure the environment so familiar tasks are repeated and new skills are introduced in a familiar context.

Profile: Diana

Diana is an eleven-year-old girl who resists hygiene routines. She dislikes having her face washed, which must be done a few times a day because she is a messy eater. Upon reflection, her mother realized that her approach to face washing with Diana was inconsistent and unpredictable. Usually just before going out, in the rush to leave, her mom would notice food on Diana's face, and would quickly moisten a cloth and swipe Diana's face. Diana always turned her head away and would try to push her mother away.

Her mom decided to try a new approach. She placed two Boardmaker pictures above Diana's placemat: Eat dinner; Wipe face. At the end of each meal, before leaving the table, Diana would take a face cloth and wipe her face. A small handheld mirror was available to help her check. Diana responded well to this new routine, which became a predictable expectation at every meal. She was happier to be able to manage this by herself, and to avoid her mom's sudden unpleasant swipe during a transition time.

Sensory Diet

When sensory processing difficulties have been identified in a child, and specific sensory strategies have been found to be helpful for that child, a "sensory diet" may be recommended. A sensory diet means providing the type, frequency, and intensity of sensory input that the child needs to maintain a calm, alert, and organized nervous system (86). Some of the activities described above may become part of a sensory diet for a child. *A sensory diet is developed individually for each child, to meet his or her specific sensory needs.* It is not a "recipe" approach, nor is it simply adding more stimulation.

A sensory diet is usually designed by an occupational or physical therapist who has done a thorough observation and assessment of your child's sensory needs. A sensory diet includes these elements:

- building sensory activities right into the daily routine;
- doing specific sensory activities (such as the Wilbargar protocol, discussed below);
- adapting the environment to include opportunities for the necessary sensory input;
- adapting your approach to the child to respect his sensory needs.

An occupational or physical therapist trained in sensory integration/sensory processing usually sets up a sensory diet or at least consults when it is being set up. National physical therapy and occupational therapy organizations (listed in the Resources section) can provide guidance in finding a PT or OT with this type of training.

Sometimes the *Wilbargar Deep Pressure and Proprioceptive Technique* is incorporated into a sensory diet. This method is designed to reduce the effects of overresponsiveness (or "sensory defensiveness") in children and adults (86). It involves providing deep pressure to the skin of the arms, back, and legs at regular intervals throughout the day, using a special therapressure brush, followed by joint compressions. Joint compression involves applying pressure through the bones into a joint. The protocol was developed by Patricia Wilbargar, an occupational therapist, and is based on sensory integration theory.

Although there have been many anecdotal reports of improvements in children with sensory processing disorder using the Wilbargar technique, it has not been studied in children with Down syndrome who are overresponsive to sensory input. Be sure to consult with an occupational or physical therapist who is trained in this technique before initiating such a protocol with your child. There are specific procedures that must be followed when using this protocol.

Profile: Andy

Andy, age fourteen, has a long bus ride to school every morning. He has to wake up early to catch the bus, and he is usually still sleepy as his mom prods him through the morning routine. By the end of the long bus ride, he is either asleep or very groggy. Andy can't get off the bus, walk into the classroom, and immediately focus on academic work. It takes him a long time to "get going" at school. Rather than having Andy come in and sit at his desk right away, his teacher has built a few routines into his arrival. First, he takes a pile of his classmates' workbooks from the teachers' desk and distributes them. Then he carries the attendance (put into a heavy binder) to the office. The teacher leaves one blackboard uncleaned from the day before so Andy can brush and wash it in the morning. These movement activities help Andy to become more alert so he will be more likely to be able to focus on his school work. He also keeps a water bottle with ice cold water on his desk while working. Cold drinks help us stay awake and alert (not to mention well hydrated!).

Sensory Strategies: Adapting the Environment

In Chapter 1 I discussed adapting the environment to provide more opportunities for trying out and practicing fine motor skills. The same principle applies in sensory processing: we can adapt the environment to accommodate our child's sensory needs and to provide the kinds of sensory input that help him be more organized. If he craves deep pressure through his jaw and is constantly picking up things and chewing on them, we can put a small container with a few oral-motor toys in each room, so that they are readily available to him. Examples might be a nubbed baby toothbrush, a textured chewing toy, gum (if he is old enough), and a whistle or blowing toy. If he is overly sensitive to certain sounds, such as the telephone ring, we can try to have a phone with an adjustable ring volume. Many of the ideas given in the sensory strategies chart are examples of adapting the environment.

Our children seem to do best in environments with consistency, structure, and clear communication of expectations. This is certainly true for all young children, but it is especially true for children with developmental and learning disabilities. Because children with Down syndrome have less flexible nervous systems and delays in learning to problem solve and adjust their reactions, many seem to respond more dramatically to small changes in their environments. As discussed below, they may have difficulty with transitions and with unexpected changes in routine.

As children with Down syndrome grow up, enter, and pass through adolescence into adulthood, they often develop patterns of behavior that they rely on to make their lives predictable and manageable. For example, when Sarah was in high school, she took a bus home every day. She then had a snack and "down time." If any activity, such as an appointment, changed that routine, I had to be sure that she knew about it at least a day ahead of time, and even then she often had difficulty adjusting to the change. Even now that she is an adult, unexpectedly changing the routine and placing different expectations on her never has a positive result.

Drs. Dennis McGuire and Brian Chicoine call this need for repetition, order, and sameness "the groove" (50). Having grooves seems to help adults with Down syndrome maintain some control over their lives and can relieve some of the stress of the overwhelming world. We can run into problems with grooves when the person becomes very fixed and inflexible in his routines and is unable to accommodate any occurrence out of the ordinary. The next section offers some strategies to help your child through transitions in a way that respects his need for grooves.

Transitions

Many young children have difficulty with transitions—that is, with stopping one activity and moving on to the next. When you tell your child to pick up his toys and come to the table for lunch, you are asking him to make a transition. Obviously, there are many transitions to be made throughout the day, and if your child resists each transition, it can lead to frustration for parents and teachers. There are many possible reasons or combinations of reasons for a child with Down syndrome to have difficulty making transitions. Here are some common ones:

- difficulty with self-regulation: it may be difficult for your child to change his level of activity and alertness quickly in order to meet the expectations of the next activity;
- difficulty both processing the instruction or request and understanding the nature of the next activity and what is expected of him;
- difficulty communicating and making himself understood;
- inconsistent, unpredictable, or inappropriate expectations of the child;
- confusion due to too many people telling him what to do;
- reluctance to stop doing an activity he is currently enjoying doing;
- dislike of the next activity.

Making Transitions Easier

Here are some tips on making transitions go more smoothly for your child. These ideas involve a combination of sensory, behavioral, and cognitive approaches.

1. Use a picture schedule to help make the day more predictable, and, therefore, more manageable for your child. Often, Picture Communication Symbols© from the Boardmaker software by

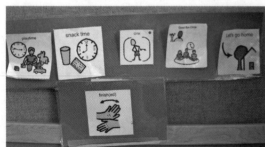

An example of a visual schedule for a preschool program, using Picture Communication Symbols© from Mayer-Johnson's Boardmaker™ software.

Mayer-Johnson are placed on a strip, showing a clear sequence of activities to help the child understand and remember the schedule. (Pictures can be arranged in a left-to-right or top-to-bottom sequence.) These pictures are particularly useful for children who have a) difficulty understanding all that is said to them, and/or b) difficulty expressing themselves verbally. For example, a child can see from a series of pictures that first he goes with Dad to pick up his sister, then he comes home and has lunch, and then he plays until naptime. He then has a sense of the sequence of activities and knows what to expect.

2. To prepare your child for a transition coming up, give him a warning such as "in five minutes we have to put on our coats and go to pick up your sister." A visual cue, such as a picture card or the picture schedule showing what is next, and/or an auditory cue such

as a timer going off can also be helpful. "Five minutes" is an abstract concept that many children do not understand. A Time Timer (timetimer.com), which is a visual timer with a red disc that gets smaller as time elapses, can be very helpful to prepare children for transitions and to help them understand the concept of time.

3. Be clear about your expectations. Help your child understand the steps of the process. Saying, "Now we're going to get your sister" may not be enough. He may need to hear the steps and see them on a visual schedule: "Now we have to stop what we're doing (wait for him to stop), put on our coats, and go in the car to get your sister."

4. In spite of all your preparations, it still may be hard for your child to leave what he is doing. Let him bring something from that activity with him to the next, such as bringing a small toy with him in the car.

5. Sometimes if a child feels he has an important role to play in the next activity, he will be more interested in stopping what he is doing and moving on. Try to find something that he likes doing. For example, perhaps he likes fastening seatbelts in the car. He can fasten his sister's and his own seatbelt so that he feels he has a helpful role to play.

6. Children can manage transitions better if they are calm and alert. If a child with poor self-regulation is overresponsive or underresponsive at that particular time, he may not be able to make the transition on his own. You may need to plan an extra few minutes into the routine to help him calm down or "rev up." To calm down your child, you may want to try one of these suggestions:

   - Join him in his activity or play, match his energy level, and gradually try to lower his energy level with your actions and voice (gradually slow down your movements and lower your voice level).
   - As he begins to calm down, a slow, rhythmic song accompanied by rhythmic actions may help him regulate himself to make the transition.

If your child can't seem to make the transition because he needs more energy (he needs to "rev up"), here are some ideas:

   - Join him in his activity or play at his energy level and gradually increase your own energy level and animation, encouraging him to join in active rhymes or songs that encourage more physical activity.
   - Light touch can bring up a person's level of alertness. Try nonthreatening touch, like gently stroking your child's fin-

gers, blowing on his hair, or touching his ears. Quick, brisk touch is also alerting, such as giving high fives and clapping.

7. Social stories (developed by Carol Gray for use with children with autism) are sometimes used to help a child understand a social situation or skill. The story describes the situation and provides examples of appropriate behavior from the perspective of those involved. It is written in a specific format (e.g., in the first person). Some children respond well to social stories and may become less resistant to transitions and other behavioral expectations.

8. There may be times when none of the above works, and you may have to resort to the Distract and Entertain routine. Take the focus off what you want him to do and put the focus on the two of you interacting through singing, acting silly, putting on a funny voice, etc., and before he knows it, he will have cooperated with what you wanted him to do!

Alertness and Self-Regulation

There are many ways we help ourselves through the day using sensory strategies without really thinking about them in that way. If we are getting drowsy on a long drive, we may turn on some loud music, chew gum, or sing to keep ourselves awake and alert. If we don't like the feel of wool on our skin, we simply don't buy wool clothing. The difference for our children is that they may not be able to identify what is making them uncomfortable or inattentive, or they may not be able to articulate it to us.

The first step for parents and teachers is to recognize that sensory input may be playing a role in your child's responses. If certain sensory inputs seem to cause your child to become more disorganized, you need to try to reduce or eliminate those from his environment. If you find other sensory inputs that help your child be more calm and organized, try to build those into his day on a regular basis. Just as fine motor activities can be incorporated into everyday routines, sensory strategies and activities can become part of your child's daily routine. Sensory strategies don't just help children with a sensory processing disorder; they help us all. Your child with Down syndrome may not have sensory processing issues, but he may still benefit from the use of sensory strategies in his daily routines.

We all respond best to environmental demands when we are in a calm, alert state. Our "state" refers to how responsive we are at that particular time to what is going on around us. Our state is also referred to as our "level of alertness." We experience a broad range of alertness levels: from sleep all the way to the heightened state of awareness and responsiveness experienced in dangerous situations.

Sensory processing helps us to change our state as necessary for the time of day and the activity we are involved in. For example, if your child is having speech therapy, he needs to be alert and attentive to the speech-language pathologist to benefit from the therapy. If he is drowsy and inattentive or overstimulated and excited, he is unlikely to get much out of the session. Many, if not most, young children need help learning how to regulate their state to the demands of their day. The bedtime routines we establish for our children can help them calm down gradually so that they will be able to fall asleep. For children who have developmental delays, medical concerns, sensory impairments, and/or sensory processing difficulties, maintaining an appropriate state throughout the day can be a challenge.

We all go through many levels of alertness throughout the day: drowsy first thing in the morning and at night, awake and responsive during normal daily activities, high level of alertness during a challenging sports activity, drowsy during a boring mid-afternoon lecture, etc. Our level of alertness is influenced by many internal and external factors. Fatigue, hunger, and physical activity level are internal factors. Medical conditions are also important factors that can affect a child and must *always* be considered first. As mentioned earlier in this chapter, hypothyroidism, sleep apnea, respiratory infections, and dehydration are critical to monitor in children with Down syndrome. We must also pay attention to the many external factors—such as noise, visual stimuli, lighting, movement, type of food and drink, and many more—that influence the level of alertness.

Self-regulation refers to the ability to reach, maintain, and change one's optimal state (level of alertness) to match the needs of the situation (86, 83). The development of self-regulation in children also involves the development of awareness of socially approved behaviors, and the ability to modify their own behavior. For example, a child with good self-regulation would be able to play an active game of tag outside, then quickly come inside when called for dinner, sit at the table, and eat. A child with poor self-regulation may not be able to make this transition so quickly and easily, may be slow to respond, and may have difficulty settling down enough to be able to sit and eat. Knowing that it is difficult for him to change his level of alertness, he may learn to resist these transitions, especially when they are unexpected, and we may see behavior that is usually described as "stubborn." The child can then learn this behavior pattern and may persist in using it even as he matures and is able to adjust his activity level more readily.

A program called *How Does Your Engine Run? The Alert Program for Self-Regulation,* developed by occupational therapists Mary Sue Williams and Sherry Shellenberger, focuses on teaching school-aged children ways to recognize, understand, and implement sensory strategies to change and keep their energy level and alertness appropriate to their needs throughout the day (see Resources for information). *Zones of Regulation* is a curriculum based on a cognitive behavior approach that helps children learn how to self-regulate using calming techniques, cognitive strategies, and sensory supports.

Alerting and Preparing Activities for Children with Down Syndrome

Levels of alertness can be influenced by all the sensory systems, including the tactile, vestibular, and proprioceptive systems. If we are feeling lethargic and low in energy, often the best way to increase our energy level and alertness is to do a movement activity, such as getting up and going for a walk. It is the same for children with Down syndrome. Self-directed movement in itself is alerting to the nervous system. Movements that can be particularly alerting and organizing for the nervous system include 1) those that involve changing the position of the head in space (vestibular input), such as going on a swing, and 2) movements that provide deep pressure through the joints (proprioceptive input), such as jumping rope.

These types of sensory input can *temporarily* change a child's level of alertness. They also provide good preparation for the body to learn a new motor task. Participating in vestibular and proprioceptive activities prepares the nervous system for a more challenging activity, such as one that is just being learned. I have a personal example of how this works. For a long time I tried to help Sarah learn how to ride a bike the usual way: by helping her get on and put her feet on the pedals and then holding the back of the seat of the bike while she rode. However, I never seemed to be able to let go of the back of the bike, as she wasn't getting the feel of balancing the bike. Finally, I tried putting her on a tire swing at the local park (which she loved); she swung and spun around for ten or fifteen minutes. When we tried the bike after the swing, she starting catching on to the balancing of the bike right away, and I was able to let go. It seemed to me that the vestibular input helped prepare her for the more challenging task of balancing the bike. This may not work for every child, and every child may not need the input to learn to ride, but there seemed to be a correlation that worked for us.

Sometimes children with Down syndrome have difficulty with self-regulation in the context of environmental and social expectations. For example, they may seem lethargic and relatively unresponsive in the classroom, only to quickly become overexcited during a social interactive game. If there is physical contact in the game, they may overdo it, grabbing and holding the other children inappropriately. The adults watching aren't sure how to respond. They are glad that the child is finally interacting with the other children, but the child's difficulties understanding social protocol and regulating his interactions are limiting his success with the others. It seems that the child's "window" of optimal alertness and responsiveness is small and that he is more often under or over the optimum level. Because of the child's cognitive delays and difficulty reading social cues and responding accordingly, using a combination of sensory strategies and behavioral approaches will probably be most helpful.

Profile: James

James is a twelve-year-old boy integrated into a regular classroom. Although quiet and somewhat noninteractive with his peers in the classroom, he "comes alive" at recess, running around randomly and trying to join games that are already going on in the schoolyard. Because he is moving around from group to group and doesn't understand the rules of the game, he causes disruption, and the other kids don't want him to join.

Recently, his teacher has recognized his need for structured movement activities with heavy work input (proprioception) to help him be more organized in his play during recess. She organized a group of eighth grade students to set up a few activities to start off recess for James and some of his classmates. They begin with a tug-of-war on the lawn and then play a game of dodge ball with a larger inflated ball (so the kids won't get hurt by the ball). They follow this up with a game of shadow tag (the kids step on each other's shadow to "catch" them in tag), so there is no reaching, touching, and grabbing, which is hard for James to both tolerate and initiate appropriately. James becomes more organized during these activities, and is more alert and interactive afterward in the classroom.

Technology

There are many apps that are described under a "Sensory" heading on app lists. Many of these apps provide simple, calming visual and/or auditory input that may help some children to maintain a calm, organized state. The *Time Timer,* mentioned above in the section on transitions, is available as an app, as are some similar products. There are also several apps that provide templates and visual options for preparing visual schedules and social stories.

GestureTek, video gesture control technology, responds to movement by changing, moving, video patterns (often projected onto a floor). I have seen many children become more animated, mobile, and interactive when engaged with this technology.

It is beyond the scope of this book to list even a small sampling of the apps that might be helpful for children, teens, and adults who have difficulties with sensory processing. However, there are many websites that list and categorize useful apps for people with disabilities. Some of these are listed in the Resources at the end of the book.

Snoezelen

Snoezelen is a concept that was developed by occupational therapists in Holland. Snoezelen is a sensory environment that provides people with severe disabilities the opportunity to enjoy and control a variety of sensory experiences. Snoezelen is usually set up as a room or part of a room, and usually includes a variety of visual lighting effects (such as a bubble tube, fiber optics, and a solar projector), soft sounds, and comfortable cushions, and it sometimes includes movement (such as a hammock), vibration, mirrors, and tactile activities. Some of the sensory experiences are soothing, while others are stimulating. Only those experiences that are appropriate for the individual's needs should be used.

Research into the effects of Snoezelen on people with challenging conditions supports the findings that it can have a positive impact on mood, behavior, and relationships. These changes are seen over time, as the child or adult

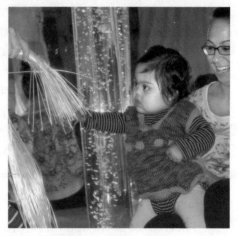

spends time regularly in the Snoezelen room, and is free to enjoy and control the sensory experience without any expectations to perform or respond in any particular way. The white rooms, which have white floors and wall mats, can be calming and organizing and can help offset some of the more demanding aspects of a person's day.

Snoezelen rooms are now available in some clinics, hospitals, schools, and residential and other facilities that serve individuals with developmental and physical disabilities.

Supplies are available through Flaghouse. (See Resources.)

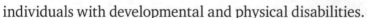

Down Syndrome and Autism Spectrum Disorders

Rates of autism spectrum disorders (ASD) have been increasing in the general population in the past ten or fifteen years. At the same time, the recognition that ASD can occur in people with Down syndrome has also been increasing. Researchers have reported different rates of co-occurring Down syndrome and autism, ranging from 3 to 18 percent of people with Down syndrome. Researchers have also found that autism spectrum disorder is more common in children with Down syndrome who have greater degrees of cognitive impairment (19).

A diagnosis of ASD is based on a cluster of symptoms that fall into three areas:

- social impairments,
- communication impairments,
- repetitive stereotyped behaviors and restricted interests (10).

As the diagnosis relies partially on delays in social and communication skills, these areas of development must be significantly impaired relative to a child's cognitive level in order for ASD to be diagnosed in a child with Down syndrome. Although many children with Down syndrome have delays in communication skills, they generally have what is called "communicative intent"—they want to communicate with others, even though they may have trouble speaking. When a child with Down syndrome also has ASD, this communicative intent is often lacking.

Some of the other signs that are sometimes seen in a child who has both Down syndrome and ASD include the following:

- decreased or no eye contact
- repetitive, self-stimulatory behaviors, such as spinning, rocking, or head banging
- seeking visual input by staring at lights or fans, flicking fingers, or dangling toys in front of eyes
- lack of purposeful play with toys; restricted and repetitive interests
- excessive mouthing of objects
- rigidity with routines
- lack of communicative intent
- limited food preferences

This is by no means a diagnostic list, but merely a reflection of what I and other professionals have seen in children who have both diagnoses. Sometimes these behaviors are present from a young age, and sometimes they begin to appear as a slightly older child seems to lose previously gained skills and communication abilities.

Many children with ASD have sensory processing difficulties (86, 44). Thus, it is likely that children with Down syndrome who are also diagnosed with ASD will have sensory processing difficulties as well. The sensory processing difficulties associated with ASD often are related to over- or under-responsiveness to sensory input. You can try the same types of approaches for handling these problems detailed in the chart on pages 233-38. Sensory processing challenges associated with a dual diagnosis may also require evaluation and recommendations from an occupational therapist.

Behavioral Approaches

This chapter has focused on sensory processing issues in children with Down syndrome, and has described some sensory strategies to help. Sometimes when children have learned patterns of behavior over time, they are difficult to change, even if the sensory environment is adapted to meet the child's needs. The child may be using the behavior for other reasons, such as to seek attention (either positive or negative), to get or avoid a particular activity or object, or to otherwise communicate. In these cases, the child often needs intervention based on positive reinforcement of desired behaviors and structured activities that ensure his success. It is beyond the scope of this book to detail the types of behavioral interventions that can be used to help children with Down syndrome who have these needs. Psychologists, behavior therapists, child care workers, and teachers are among the professionals who develop and carry out programs based on behavioral principles.

Summary

Our ability to interact adaptively with our environment depends partly on the sensory information available, partly on the processing and integration of that sensory information, and partly on our own unique personality and genetic makeup. When faced with puzzling behaviors in our children with Down syndrome, we must first rule out intrinsic factors such as medical conditions, hunger, thirst, fatigue, illness, communication difficulties, and visual or hearing problem. When these are ruled out or managed, we can consider how the sensory environment may be contributing to the child's problematic responses, and what we might be able to change in the sensory environment to help him behave more appropriately.

If your child *overreacts* to certain types of sensory input (light touch and certain sounds are the most common), you can try to change the environment to reduce these types of input *and* provide deep pressure and proprioceptive input throughout the day.

If your child *underreacts* to certain types of sensory input, you can try to enrich his environment with the types of sensory input you have noticed help him to become more aware and alert (visual, touch, and movement inputs are the most common).

If your child seeks sensory input beyond what is expected for his developmental age, you can try to provide regular opportunities for sensory input through various sensory channels (i.e., a sensory diet) that will provide what his nervous system seeks, without overstimulating him.

If your child doesn't seem to overreact or underreact but has a lot of difficulty organizing movement and learning new movement skills, you can ensure that he has an environment rich in tactile exploration and body awareness activities. You can also use verbal and visual feedback to help him.

As a parent, you can take note of environments that help your child be most interactive, calm, attentive, and happy. We can also take note of environments that lead to more anxiety and disorganized or disruptive responses. Sometimes you may see patterns in the way your child processes sensory information that indicate sensory needs or avoidances. Sometimes you can sort this out yourself and reach solutions that improve your child's situation. Other times you may need the assistance of an occupational therapist or physical therapist trained in sensory integration/sensory processing. Remember: if there is not a pattern that seems to fit a sensory perspective, your child may be responding to other needs, such as the need for attention, the need to communicate, etc. You can consult with speech-language pathologists, psychologists, behavior therapists, teachers, and other medical and educational professionals for help with your child's challenging behaviors.

Grandma's and Grandpa's List

- Hop balls
- Inflatable punching bag
- Parachute
- Tether ball
- Beanbag chair
- Hammock
- Rocking horse
- Rocker/balance/"wobble" board
- Air mattress
- Ball pool
- Cloth crawl tunnels
- Vibrating stuffed toy
- Sit 'n Spin
- Fidget toys (small handheld toys that can be manipulated and/or have a pleasing sensory property, such as a bumpy surface. Twiddle Fidget crunch shape is an example)
- Foam floor mats
- Balance bike (no pedals)
- Plasmacar
- Boardmaker software (Mayer-Johnson)
- Visual schedule apps; First-then apps
- Time Timer
- Move 'n Sit cushion

12

Hands Up!

You've gotta dance like there's nobody watching, love like you'll never be hurt,
sing like there's nobody listening, and live like it's heaven on earth.
—William W. Purkey

We can all take a lesson from the book on "how to live a life" by people who have Down syndrome. If you haven't read "If People with Down Syndrome Ruled the World" by Dennis McGuire, look it up online and read it. It is a refreshingly honest take on living life with someone who has Down syndrome.

Fine motor skills, sensory processing, independent living skills, etc., are all part of the bigger picture. Yes, there are many things we can do to facilitate the development of our children. When they are adults, there are roles for us as supports and advocates for their rights to be included in all aspects of culture and society. Everything—all the skills learned and abilities gained revolves around one thing: ***RELATIONSHIPS.***

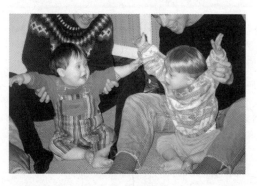

We all need a context to make life meaningful; we all need relationships. Our children with Down syndrome have a unique relationship with us, their parents, that often continues into adulthood in a codependent living relationship, whether they live with us or not. Relationships within the family, extended family, and in the community are vitally important to our children, and must be nurtured.

Our society is driven by the motivations and aspirations of the individual, by success, and by financial security. Our children with Down syndrome do not necessarily fit into this mold; they challenge us and all those in contact with them to develop new expectations of life. Our challenge as parents may not be so much to try to help our children fit into the mold, but to try to change and expand this mold, to help develop acceptance and inclusion, not just tolerance.

I hope this book can be a help to parents. I know that often I find comfort in just talking to another parent who understands what it is all about.

Appendix 1:
Visual Motor Worksheets

Workbooks and programs that have activities for tracing and copying in preparation for printing are available through most toy and educational stores. I designed some of my own for Sarah based on her interests and the types of pencil movements she would need to learn to be able to print letters and numbers. I have divided the visual motor practice into four stages.

Stage 1

These worksheets are designed for children with Down syndrome who are making simple strokes on paper. For many children with Down syndrome, these worksheets will be appropriate from about ages three to five. The worksheets can be used with different media, but the way patterns are introduced should be consistent. The marker/paintbrush/pencil should always begin at the monkey's face and then follow the pattern. In all the linear patterns, show your child how to stop at the corner and change direction. For most children of this age, this will be a new concept. It is not important at this stage for your child to stay neatly within the lines. The points you want him to learn from these activities are the following:

- There is a definite starting point.
- He needs to stop his stroke to change direction.
- There is a definite stopping point.

The direction and patterns are based on some of the uppercase letter patterns that your child will learn to print. The worksheets can be enlarged and used on an easel, with your child following the pattern with his paintbrush. Or your child can take a thick crayon or marker and stroke along the pattern to fill the space with color. Your child can roll out a snake of play dough and lay it on top of the pattern or do the same with a Wikki Stix. The inverted *V* pattern will be the most difficult for most children as the monkey tells them to start at the top and draw down the left side, then pick up their marker, go back to the top, and down the other side. This exercise is included because several uppercase letters are printed in this way, returning to the starting point to begin the next stroke.

Stage 2

The next set of worksheets is for children who already have the ability to make circles and vertical and horizontal lines and have begun to combine them in simple forms. They may also be learning to print, as most children are introduced to printing their own name at about age four or five. These worksheets will help your child refine his control of the pencil in preparation for printing lowercase letters. Your child will also develop these skills: starting and stopping the stroke at a defined spot; making smaller strokes within a defined space; and controlling the direction of the stroke more precisely. These worksheets can be appropriate for ages four and up, depending on your child's level. The use of each worksheet is as follows:

- **CLOWN:** make horizontal lines across the clown's costume
- **TRAIN TRACKS:** make vertical lines across tracks; diagonal lines for crossing signs
- **PORCUPINE:** make short lines in various directions
- **HOUSE:** make a cross in each window
- **FISH:** make semicircles starting at the top and going in a counter-clockwise direction (top fish) and clockwise direction (bottom fish)
- **FISH BUBBLES:** make very small circles
- **FACES:** add eyes and mouth on each face

Stage 3

One example of how letters can be grouped to teach printing of lowercase letters is presented here. I am providing this information to help parents, teachers, and teacher assistants think about how a particular child will best learn to print using consistent patterns that will make it easier for him to remember how to form the letters. Other therapists and educators may suggest slightly different letter groupings. I don't advocate one method over another, but I do feel that children have more chances of success with printing if they are taught one method consistently, with attention to how the letters are formed. As mentioned in Chapter 9, a multisensory approach to learning letter formation can help some children.

Letter Groups:

1. a, d, g, q: These letters all begin with a curved (counterclockwise) stroke and then proceed into a vertical line. The line is retraced, continuing below the line for g and q.
2. c, o, e, s: Like group 1, these letters involve a curved stroke in a counterclockwise direction. The letters e and s are a bit different, but are included in this group because the curved stroke begins in the same direction.
3. l, t, f, k: These letters all begin with a straight vertical line down (in the case of f, it begins with a little hook and then proceeds down in a vertical line). The pencil is then lifted to make the cross stroke in t and f, and the diagonal strokes in k.
4. i, j: Like the letters in group 3, these also begin with a vertical line. The letter j ends with a little hook at the end.
5. h, b, p: These letters also begin with a vertical line down, which is then retraced partially to proceed into the curved (clockwise) stroke. The letter p is retraced back up to the top of the line.
6. n, m, r: These letters begin with a short vertical line, which is retraced up to begin the curved stroke. The middle line is also retraced in m.
7. u, v, w, x, y, z: These letters (except for z) begin with a downward stroke: u curves; v, w, and y are diagonals. The letter z includes a diagonal line but begins with a horizontal stroke.

Stage 4

The last set of worksheets provides prewriting patterns that will help children who are preparing to learn cursive writing. They cover the basic patterns of pencil movement that are found in most of the letters. Again, similar types of writing practice are available in other workbooks and programs. These worksheets are provided so that parents and teachers can photocopy them for repeated use with a child. Alternately, they can be placed in a plastic cover so that the child can practice with an erasable marker.

STAGE 1–DIAGONAL LINES (begin drawing at the monkey face)

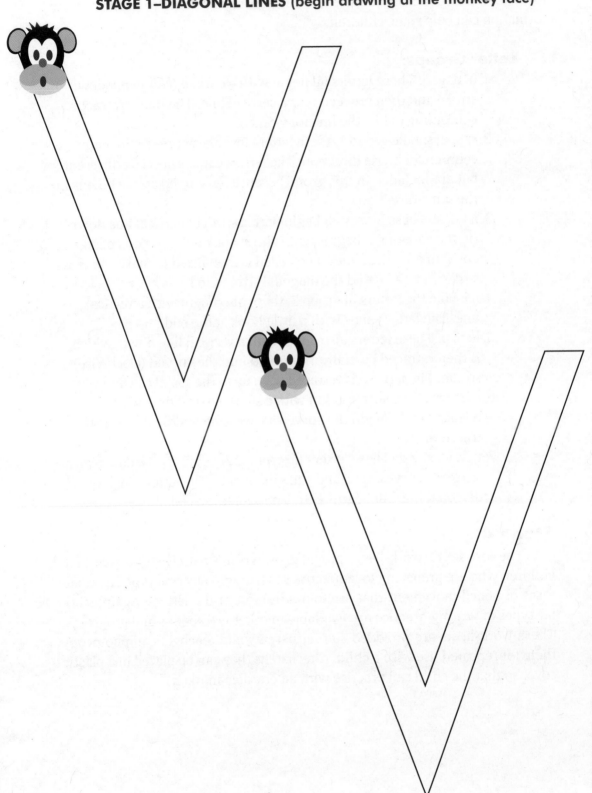

STAGE 1—CIRCLES (begin drawing at the monkey face)

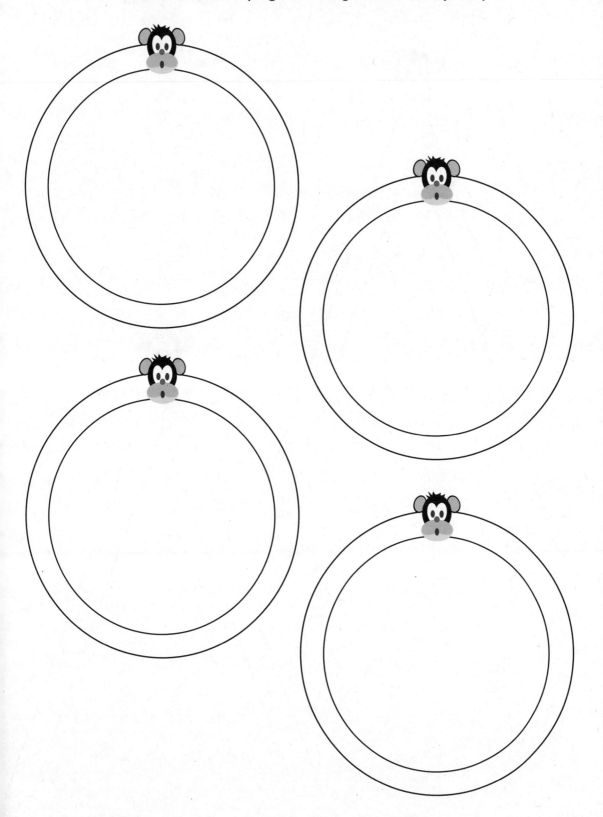

STAGE 1–DIAGONAL LINES (begin drawing at monkey face)

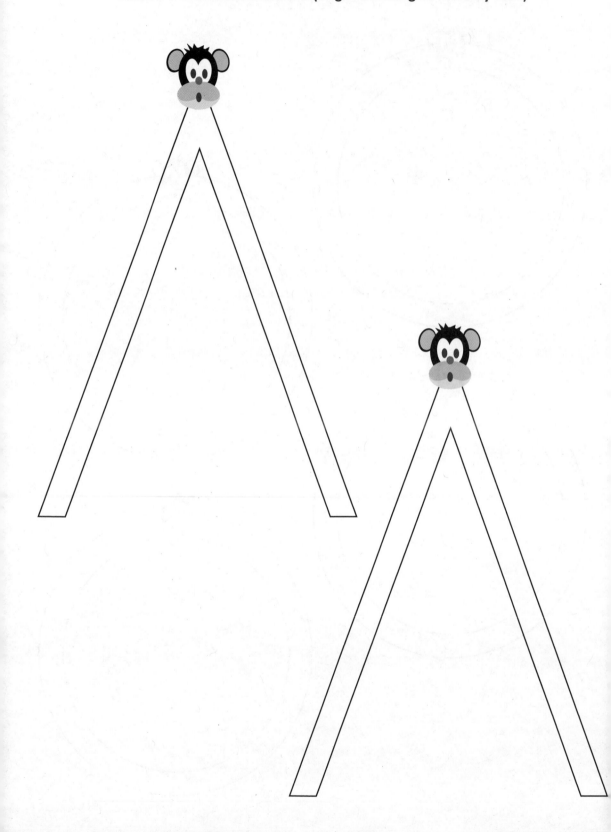

STAGE 1–STRAIGHT LINES (begin drawing at monkey face)

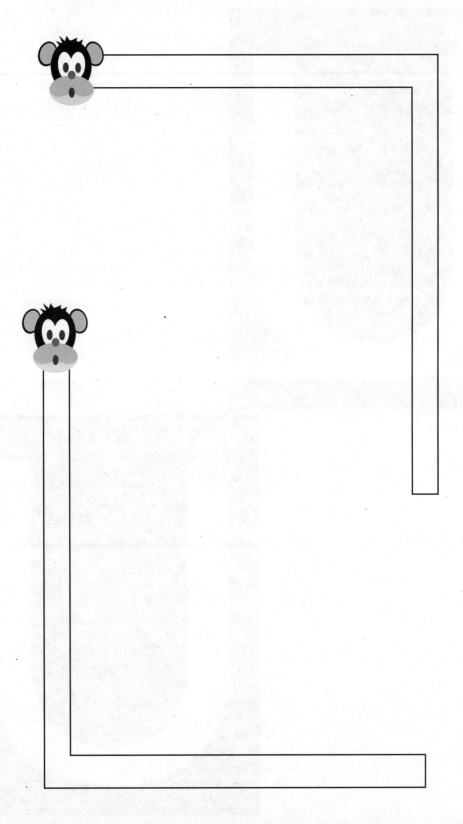

STAGE 1–CURVED (begin drawing at the monkey face)

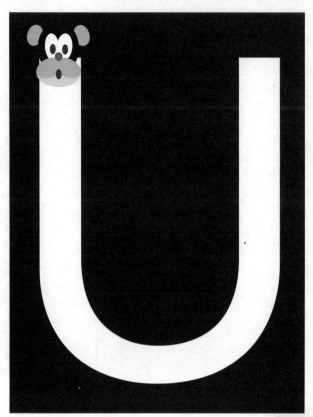

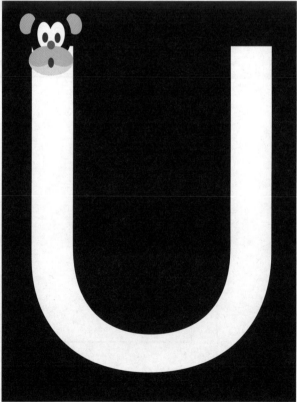

STAGE 1—CURVED LINES (begin drawing at the monkey face)

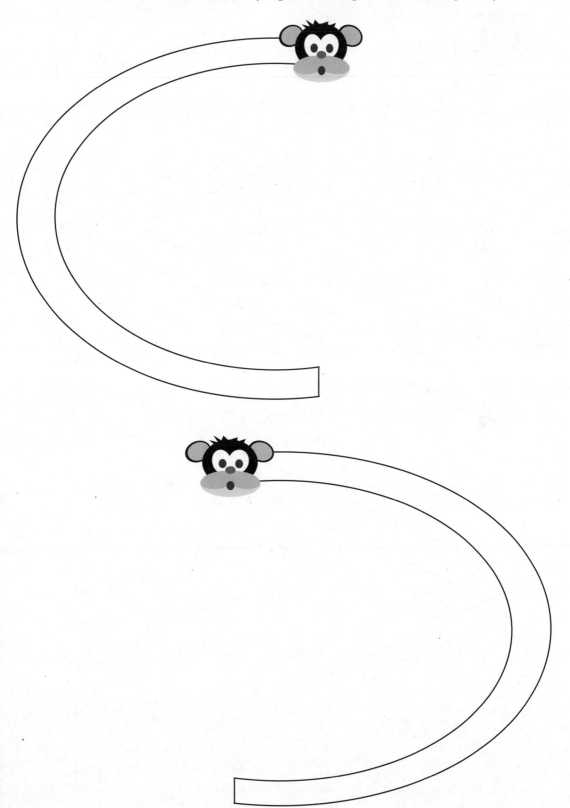

STAGE 1–DIAGONAL LINES (begin drawing at the monkey face)

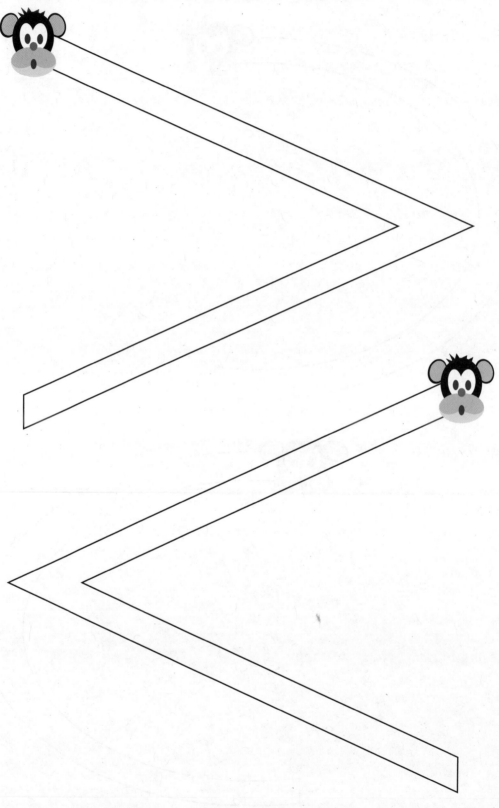

stage 2–clown (draw horizontal lines)

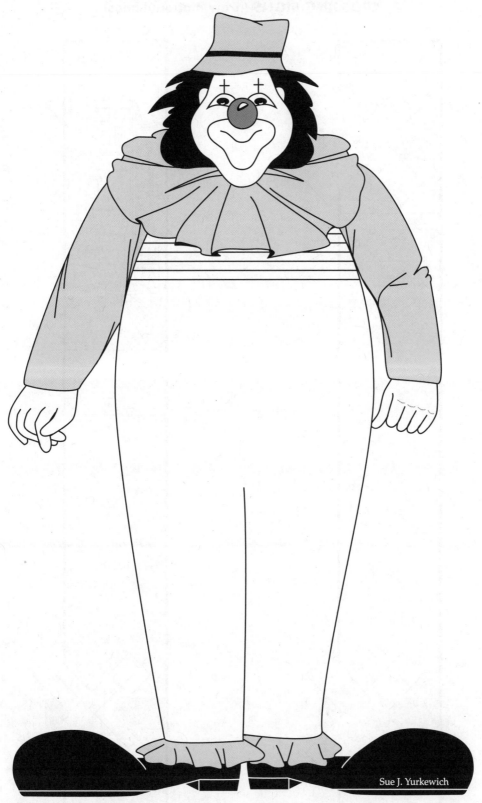

Sue J. Yurkewich

STAGE 2–TRAIN TRACKS (draw vertical lines)
CROSSING SIGNS (draw diagonal lines)

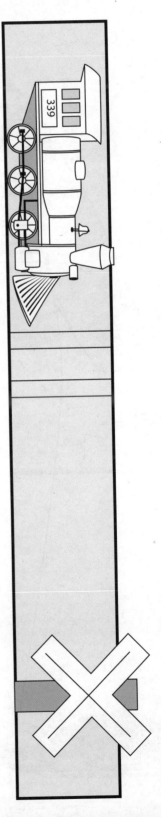

Sue J. Yurkewich

STAGE 2–PORCUPINE (draw lines various directions)

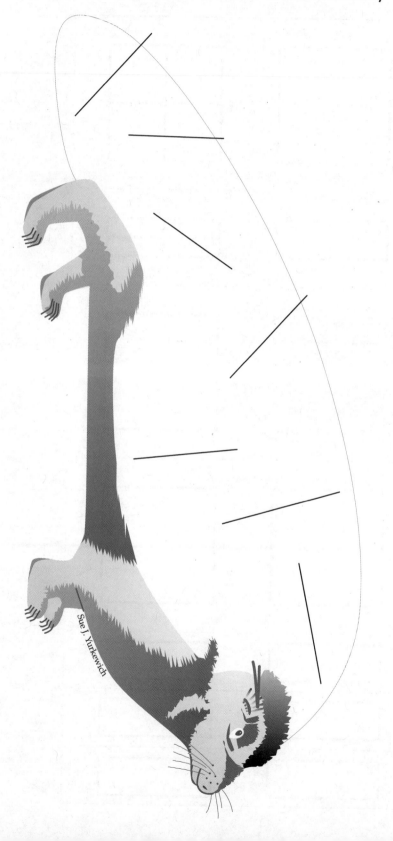

Sue J. Yurkewich

STAGE 2–HOUSE WINDOWS (draw crossing lines)

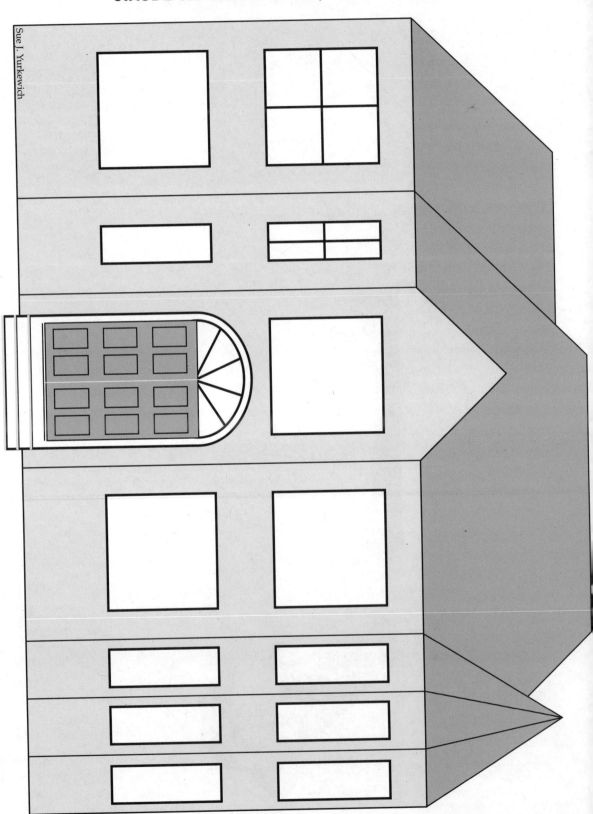

Sue J. Yurkewich

STAGE 2–FISH SCALES (draw semicircles clockwise & counterclockwise)
BUBBLES (draw small circles)

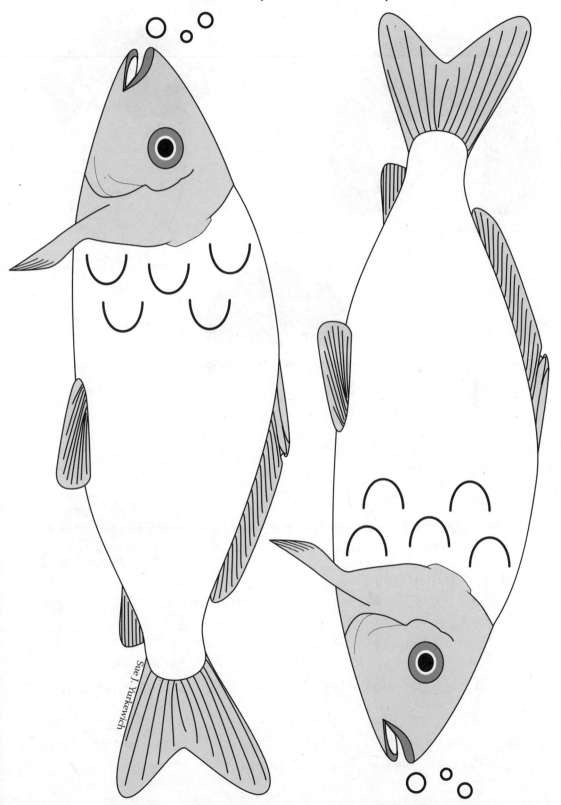

Sue J. Yurkewich

STAGE 2–FACES (draw features)

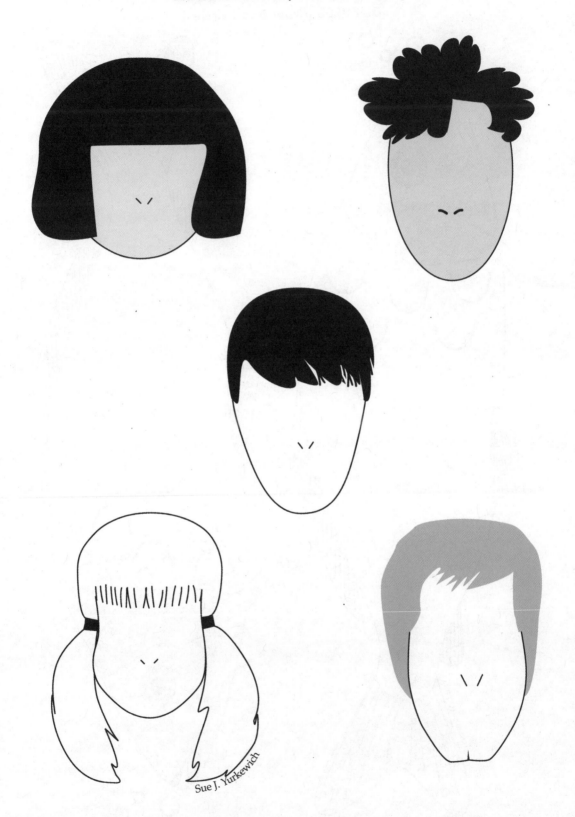

Sue J. Yurkewich

STAGE 4–ROLLER COASTER (finish the ride on the roller coaster)

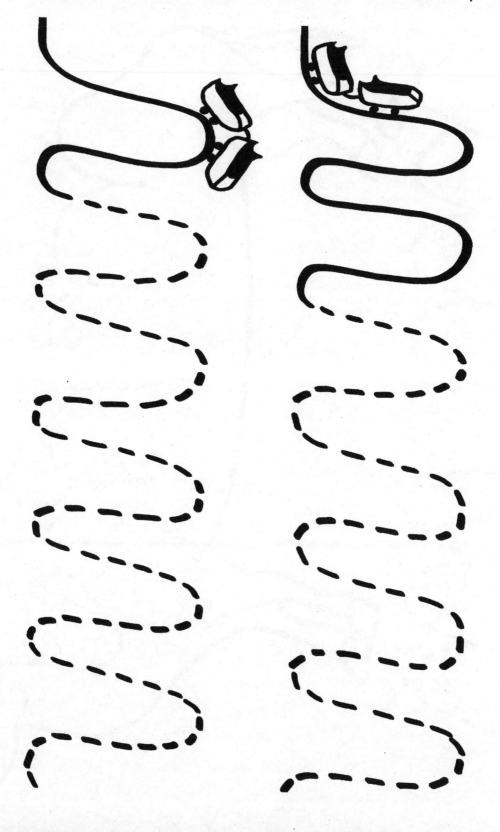

STAGE 4–CAMEL (finish the camel's humps; practice below)

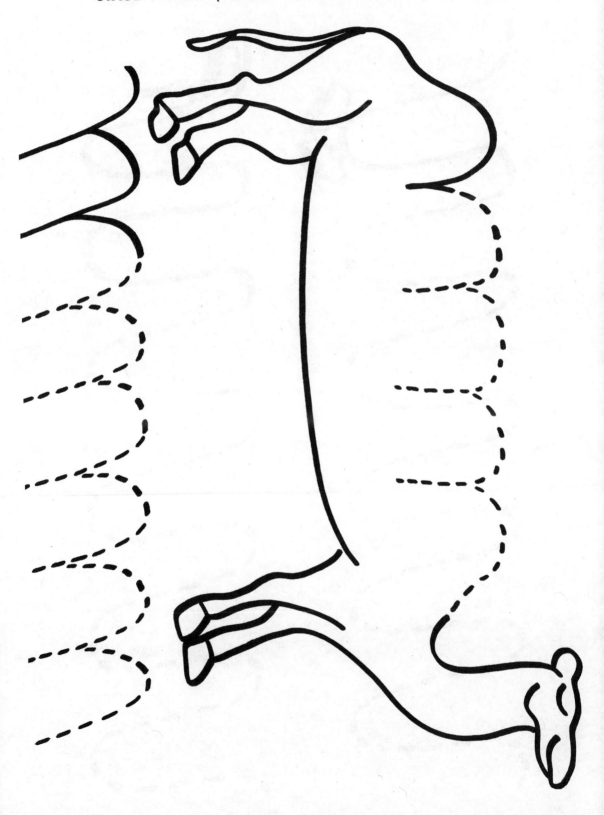

STAGE 4–SPIDER (finish the spider's walk on the tall grass)

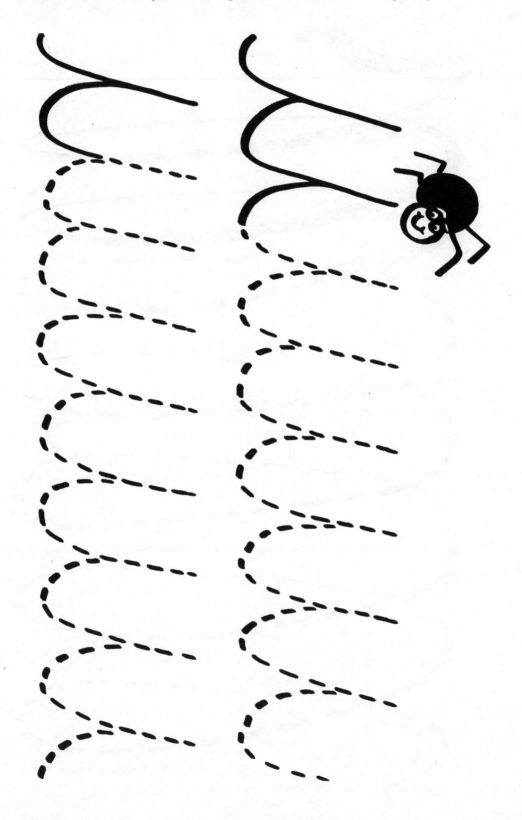

STAGE **4**–BOOMERANG (finish the boomerang's path)

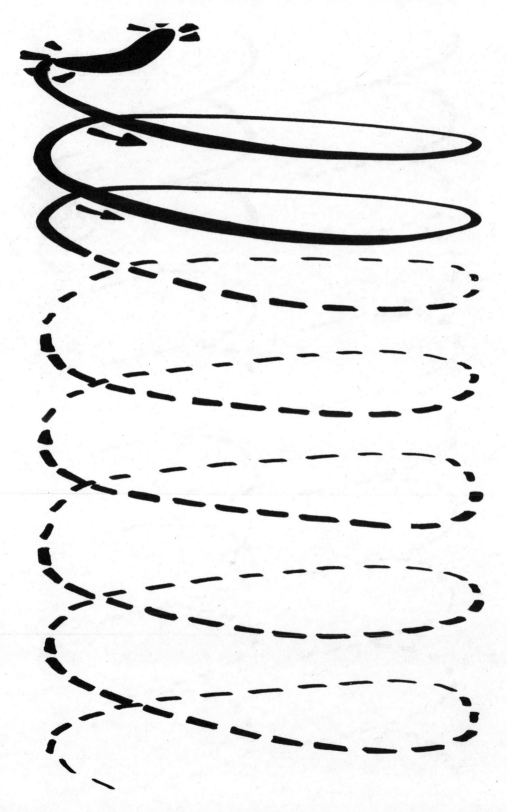

STAGE 4–BIRD (finish the bird's flight)

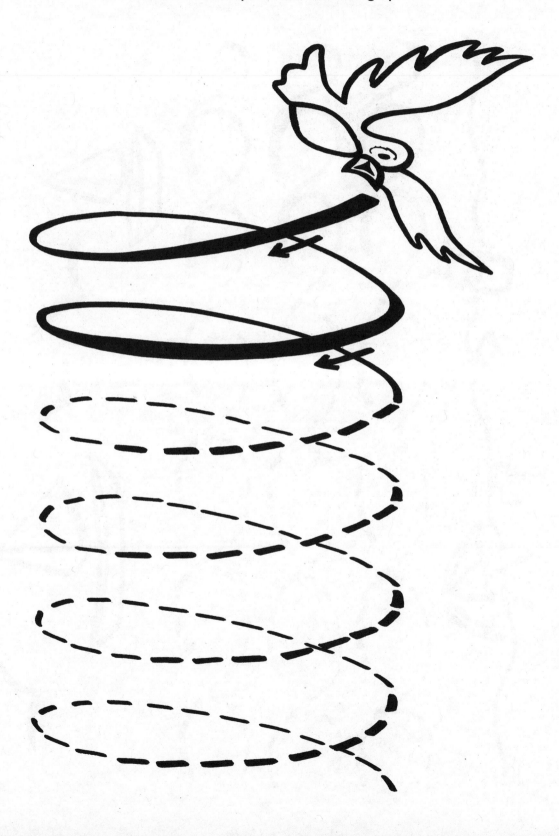

STAGE 4–WAVES (finish the waves)

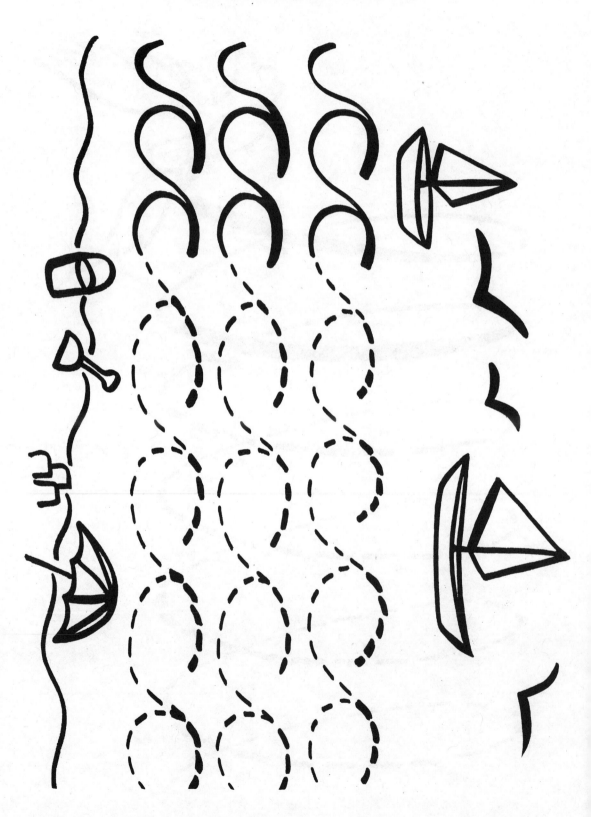

Appendix 2:
Don't Throw It Out!

S ome of the activities described in this book make use of everyday items that are around the house. Here is a list of things families often have around the house, and their uses:

- Empty plastic pop bottles: fill with colorful beads, marbles—any-thing that will make a nice noise as your child moves it around and picks it up. It's good for early bilateral hand skills, as the bottle has to be picked up with both hands.
- Empty plastic yogurt, ice cream, or other containers: cut a hole or slot in the top for dropping objects into. You can also cut out the center of the lids, leaving only the rims, to be used as rings to put on pegs (or empty paper towel rolls). Simple shapes can be cut out of a lid to make a stencil.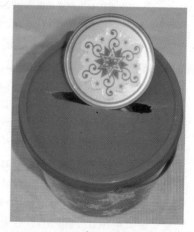
- Empty bleach containers: cut off the bottom of the container to make a "scoop catcher," which is held to catch beanbags or other tossed items.
- Paper rolls: a paper towel or toilet paper roll can be glued to a piece of cardboard and used as a peg. Put cut-out margarine con-tainer lids or bracelets on it (rings on peg game). Paper rolls can also be used for making a variety of crafts.

- Empty squeeze bottles, such as dish detergent bottles: wash out well and use in the bathtub for water play.
- Measuring cups: a set of measuring cups that fit into one another can be used for learning concepts of taking apart/putting together, and size discrimination.
- Bangle bracelets: guiding the hand through to put the bracelet on helps develop hand awareness skills for a toddler or young child.
- Empty orange juice cans (no rough edges): for paints; filling and pouring water activities; stacking.

- Tennis ball containers: cut holes and slots in lids and have the child put in ping pong balls, dowels, etc.
- Pots and pans: a favorite of all toddlers—practice taking lids on and off, stirring with a wooden spoon, etc.
- Dried-up markers: still good for pulling the caps on and off. Improvise a pegboard by cutting holes in a block of Styrofoam that the markers can stand up in.
- Plastic "bubble" wrapping paper: use it for a different sensory experience or to develop pinch strength when trying to pop the bubbles. Supervise closely; it is plastic!
- Cardboard boxes: use larger, sturdy boxes as sitting stools, footstools, or as "tables" for children playing on the floor (cut out a semicircle for their legs). This may help the child who is just becoming independent in sitting by raising the height of the toys.
- Shoeboxes: use as large building blocks.
- Tissue paper: great for ripping or cutting into small pieces, scrunching into a ball, and gluing on paper.
- Single socks or mittens: sew on buttons or wool to make hand puppets with funny faces, or make beanbags out of them.
- Buttons: can be used to practice picking up and releasing small objects and also for making crafts. Only for children who no longer put things in their mouth!
- Scarves: an old scarf has many uses, such as playing peek-a-boo, waving in the air to music, wrapping up small objects, etc. You can also cut very small holes in the sides of a cardboard box, put a scarf through the hole with a large bead tied to the end. Make sure the holes are small enough so that the child grasps the bead

and has to use some hand strength to pull on the scarf.
■ Coffee cans with lids can be used as tom-toms (drums).
■ Magazines, calendars: use to practice cutting out pictures.

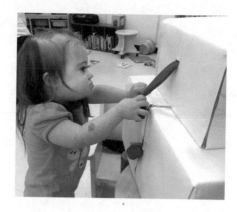

Glossary

Here is a brief compilation of terms you may encounter in this book or in your contacts with various professionals involved with your child.

app—short for "application." A software program that can be downloaded onto a device such as a phone or iPad.

arches—the contours of the palm of the hand that position the hand for function.

assistive technology—a piece of equipment or system that is used to increase, maintain, or improve functional capabilities of persons with disabilities.

asymmetrical—one side of the body is positioned or is moving differently from the other side.

atlanto-axial instability—excessive movement at the junction between the two top bones of the spine, the atlas (C1) and axis (C2), as a result of either a bony or ligamentous abnormality.

atlanto-occipital instability—excessive movement at the junction of the atlas (the top bone of the spine) and occipital bones (back part of the skull).

bilateral—relating to both hands, or both sides of the body.

camptodactyly—a permanent bent (flexed) position of one or both of the small joints of a finger, usually the fifth finger in Down syndrome.

cause-effect—(in reference to toys) the concept that something happens when the child activates the toy (e.g., a jack-in-the box is a cause-effect toy).

clinodactyly—a permanent curving inward of a finger. Usually the fifth finger in Down syndrome.

dexterity—the ability to make accurate and efficient hand movements.

digital-pronate grasp—a grasp used to hold a pencil or tool handle in which the shaft or handle is stabilized in the palm, while the thumb and second and third finger extend to the end; the second stage of grasp development.

distal—referring to the parts of the body that are furthest from the center of the body (e.g., the hands and feet are distal in the body). The opposite of *proximal.*

dominance—referring to the hand used for most activities; i.e., right-handed or left-handed.

extension—a movement of a joint, usually straightening it (e.g., elbow extension occurs when the elbow is straight). The opposite of *flexion.*

facilitate—to help something to happen.

flexion—a movement of a joint, usually bending it so that the two long bones come closer together. The opposite of *extension.*

forearm—the part of the arm between the elbow and the wrist.

hyperextension—straightening of the joint beyond the normal limits (sometimes referred to as being "double-jointed").

hypotonia—the condition in which muscles don't have the normal amount of tone, or contraction, so they appear loose and floppy. Also referred to as *low muscle tone.*

joint—the point where two or more bones meet, usually where movement occurs.

kinesthesia/kinesthetic—the sense of one's body in space; knowing where all one's body parts are in relation to each other.

laterality—refers to one side of the body or brain.

ligamentous laxity—loose ligaments around a joint, allowing it to move more then the normal amount.

low muscle tone—see hypotonia.

manipulation—the use of the hands to perform any function.

midline—the middle or center of the body in the vertical plane (e.g., the hands are in the midline when they come together in a prayer position).

muscle tone—the degree of contraction or firmness of muscles.

neurodevelopment therapy (NDT)—therapy involving handling and positioning of the child to facilitate normal postural reactions and movement patterns.

opposition—the thumb and one fingertip coming together.

palmar digital grasp—see digital-pronate grasp.

palmar grasp—a grasp in which the utensil or pencil is held firmly in the palm by all the fingers and thumb; the first stage of grasp development.

peer—a child of the same age as a given child.

pincer grasp—the thumb and first finger come together to pick up small objects; *inferior pincer* refers to the pad of the thumb opposing the side or pad of the index finger; *superior pincer* refers to the tip of the thumb opposing the tip of the index finger.

prehension—the movement of grasping, or taking hold of something.

productive skills—activity done for a specific purpose; e.g., work and housework for adults; school for children.

pronation—(related to fine motor skills) the normal resting position of the forearms and hands (palms down); the opposite of *supination.*

proprioception—the sense of position and movement that we receive from the sensors in our muscles, tendons, and joints.

proximal—the parts of the body closest to the center of the body; the opposite of distal, e.g., the shoulders are proximal and the hands are distal.

quadruped grasp—a grasp used to hold a pencil or utensil, in which the shaft or handle rests between the thumb and three fingers; a variation of the tripod grasp.

reflex—an involuntary movement or action; e.g., a cough when something is stuck in one's throat is a reflex. Many early movements in babies are reflexes; e.g., the grasp reflex occurs when an object is placed in an infant's palm.

sensory/sensation—information available to use through our senses of sight, hearing, smell, taste, touch, kinesthesia, proprioception, and vestibular. Sensory activites use touch and movement to give sensory information.

sensory integration—the neurological process that enables us to organize and integrate sensations from our body and the environment so that we can make an adaptive response.

sensory processing—the neurological process of registering, orienting to, modulating, interpreting, and integrating sensory information from our body and the environment in order to make an adaptive response.

stability—the ability to hold steady; stability of muscles forms a foundation and base upon which movement can occur.

storing—keeping small items tucked into the palm of the hand.

supination—(related to fine motor skills) rotating the wrist to turn the forearm and the palm up; opposite of *pronation.*

symmetrical—the two sides of the body are equal; positioned or moving in the same way.

transfer—to pass an object from one hand to the other.

transference—moving an object from the palm out to the fingers.

tripod grasp—a grasp used to hold an object, pencil, or handle in which the thumb and second and third fingers hold the object out of the palm. *Static tripod* refers to a pencil grasp in which the shaft rests between the pads of the thumb and second and third fingers and most of the movement comes from the wrist, elbow, and shoulder. *Dynamic tripod* refers to a pencil grasp in which the shaft rests between the tips of the thumb, which is rounded, and the second and third fingers, where the movement comes from the small joints of the fingers and thumb.

vestibular system—the sensory system located in the inner ear that subconsciously informs us about movement and head position and helps us maintain an upright posture.

visual motor—refers to activities in which the eyes guide hand movement (e.g., printing, drawing).

voluntary movement—moving with intention; the opposite of *reflex*.

Bibliography

Included in this bibliography are all the books and articles I researched while writing this book. Some are cited in the text, as indicated by a bracketed number in the text. Others, such as those related to self-help skills, development, and handwriting programs, are included because they may be of interest to parents.

1. Anson, J. Greg . "Neuromotor Control and Down Syndrome." *Approaches to the Study of Motor Control and Learning,* edited by J. J. Summers, 387–411. Amsterdam: North-Holland, 1992.

2. Baker, Bruce L., and Alan J. Brightman. *Steps to Independence: Teaching Everyday Skills to Children with Special Needs.* 4th edition. Baltimore, MD: Paul H. Brookes, 2003.

3. Benbow, Mary. *Neurokinesthetic Approach to Hand Function and Handwriting.* Corning, NY: Advanced Rehabilitation Institutes, 1994.

4. Black, Bob. "Educational Software for Children with Down Syndrome: An Update." *Down Syndrome News and Update* 6, no. 2 (2006): 66–68.

5. Blanche, Erna I., Tina M. Botticelli, and Mary K. Hallway. "The Use of Neurodevelopmental Treatment and Sensory Integration in the Assessment and Treatment of Children with Developmental Disorders: Down Syndrome." In *Combining Neuro-Developmental Treatment and Sensory Integration Principles.* San Antonio, TX: Therapy Skill Builders, 1995.

6. Block, Martin E. "Motor Development in Children with Down Syndrome: A Review of the Literature." *Adapted Physical Activity Quarterly* 8 (1991): 179–209.

7. Boehme, Regi. *Improving Upper Body Control.* San Diego: Singular Publishing Co., 1988.

8. Boehme, Regi. *The Hypotonic Child: Treatment for Postural Control, Endurance, Strength, and Sensory Organization.* Tucson: Therapy Skill Builders, 1990.

9. Bruni, M., D. Cameron, S. Dua, and S. Noy. "Reported Sensory Processing of Children with Down Syndrome." *Physical and Occupational Therapy in Pediatrics* 30, vol. 4 (2010).

10. Buckley, S. J. "Autism and Down Syndrome." *Down Syndrome News and Update* 4, no. 4 (2005): 114–120.

11. Burns, Yvonne, and Pat Gun, eds. *Down Syndrome: Moving through Life.* New York: Chapman & Hall, 1993.

12. Carr, Janet. *Down's Syndrome: Children Growing Up.* Cambridge: Cambridge University Press, 1995.

13. Cadoret, Genevieve, and Anne Beuter. "Early Development of Reaching in Down Syndrome Infants." *Early Human Development* 36 (1994): 157–73.

14. Capone, George. "Dual Diagnosis: Down Syndrome and Neurobehavioral Disorders in Children." Philadelphia: National Down Syndrome Congress Annual Convention (audiotape of presentation), 2003.

15. Cohen, Willian, Lynn Nadel, and Myra Madnick, eds. *Visions for the 21st Century: Down Syndrome.* New York: John Wiley & Sons, 2002.

16. Cole, Kelly J., James H. Abbs, and Greg S. Turner. (1988). "Deficits in the Production of Grip Forces in Down Syndrome." *Developmental Medicine and Child Neurology* 30 (1988): 752–58.

17. Connolly, B., S. Morgan, and F. F. Russell. "Evaluation of Children with Down Syndrome Who Participated in an Early Intervention Program: Second Follow-up Study." *Physical Therapy* 64 (1984): 1515–9.

18. Cuskelly, M., A. Jobling, S. Buckley, eds. *Down Syndrome Across the Life Span.* London: Whurr Publishers, 2002.

19. Diguiseppi, C. "Screening for Autism Spectrum Disorders in Children with Down Syndrome." *Journal of Developmental and Behavioral Pediatrics* 31 (2010):181–91.

20. Dunn Klein, Marsha. *Predressing Skills.* San Antonio, TX: Therapy Skill Builders, 1983.

21. Dunn Klein, Marsha. *Pre-Writing Skills.* San Antonio, TX: Therapy Skill Builders, 1982.

22. Dunn, W. (*1999*) *Sensory Profile: User's Manual.* San Antonio, TX: Psychological Association, 1999.

23. Dyer, S., P. Gunn, H. Rauh, and P. Berry. "Motor Development in Down Syndrome Children: An Analysis of the Motor Scale of the Bayley Scales of Infant Development." *Motor Development, Adapted Physical Activity and Mental Retardation* 30 (1990): 7–20.

24. Edwards, Sandra J., and Mary K. Lafreniere. "Hand Function in the Down Syndrome Population." In *Hand Function in the Child: Foundations for Remediation,* edited by Martha Sasser. St. Louis: Mosby Year Book Inc., 1995.

25. Erhardt, Rhoda P. *Developmental Prehension Assessment.* Laurel, MD: RAMSCO Publishing Co., 1982.

26. Feng, J., J. Lazar, L. Kumin, and A. Ozok. "Computer Usage by Children with Down Syndrome: Challenges and Future Research." *ACM Transactions on Accessible Computing* 3, no. 3 (March 2010): Article 13.

27. Freeman, Andrew R., Joyce R. MacKinnon, Linda T. Miler. (2004). "Assistive Technology and Handwriting Problems: What Do Occupational Therapists Recommend?" *Canadian Journal of Occupational Therapy* 3, vol. 71 (2004): 150–60.

28. Haley, Stephen M. (1986). "Postural Reactions in Infants with Down Syndrome: Relationship to Motor Milestone Development and Age." *Physical Therapy* 66, no. 1 (1986): 17–22.

29. Haley, Stephen M. (1987). "Sequence of Development of Postural Reactions by Infants with Down Syndrome." *Developmental Medicine and Child Neurology* 29, no. 5 (1987): 674–79.

30. Hannaford, Carla. *Smart Moves: Why Learning Is Not All in Your Head.* Arlington, VA: Great Ocean Publishers, 1995.

31. Hanson, Marci J. *Teaching the Infant with Down Syndrome: A Guide for Parents and Professionals.* Austin, TX: Pro-Ed, 1987.

32. Harris, Susan R. "Physical Therapy and Infants with Down's Syndrome: The Effects of Early Intervention." *Rehabilitation Literature* 42, no. 11–12 (1981).

33. Henderson, Sheila E. "Motor Skill Development." In *Current Approaches to Down's Syndrome,* edited by David Lane and Brian Stratford. New York: Praeger Special Studies, 1985.

34. Hohlstein, Rita R. "The Development of Prehension in Normal Infants." *American Journal of Occupational Therapy* 36, no. 3 (March 1982).

35. Hogg, J., and S. C. Moss. "Prehensile Development in Down's Syndrome and Non-handicapped Preschool Children." *British Journal of Developmental Psychology* 1 (1983): 189–204.

36. Janzen, Paul, Susie Blackstein-Adler, and Kim Antonius. *Cheap N Free Access Solutions for the Mac: Communication and Writing Aids.* Toronto: Bloorview McMillan Centre, 1997.

37. Jenkins J.R., R. Fewell, and S.R. Harris. (1983). "Comparison of Sensory Integrative Therapy and Motor Programming. "*American Journal of Mental Deficiency* 88, no. 2: 221–4.

38. Jobling, Anne. "Attainment of Motor Proficiency in School-Aged Children with Down Syndrome." *Adapted Physical Activity Quarterly* 16 (1999): 344–61.

39. Jobling, Anne, and Naznin Virji-Babul. *Down Syndrome: Play, Move and Grow.* Vancouver, BC: Down Syndrome Research Foundation, 2004.

40. Johnson Levine, Kristin. *Development of Pre-Academic Fine Motor Skills: A Visual Analysis.* San Antonio, TX: Therapy Skill Builders, 1994.

41. Kumin, L., J. Lazar, and J. Feng. "Expanding Job Options: Potential Computer- Related Employment for Adults with Down Syndrome." *ACMSIGACCESS Accessibility and Computing* 103 (2012): 14–23.

42. Kumin, L. *Classroom Language Skills for Children with Down Syndrome.* Bethesda, MD: Woodbine House, 2001.

43. Lane, S.J., L. J. Miller, and B. E. Hanft. "Toward a Consensus in Terminology in Sensory Integration Theory and Practice: Part 2: Sensory Integration Patterns of Function." *Sensory Integration Special Interest Section Quarterly* 23 (2000).

44. Lashno, Mary. "Observations of Children with Down Syndrome and Autistic Spectrum Disorder." *Disability Solutions* 3, no. 5–6 (1999).

45. Lashno, Mary. "Sensory Processing Disorder." Philadelphia: National Down Syndrome Congress Annual Convention (audiotape of presentation), 2003.

46. Lauteslager, P.E.M., A. Vermeer, and P. J. M. Helders. "Disturbances in the Motor Behavior of Children with Down Syndrome: The Need for a Theoretical Framework." *Physiotherapy* 84, no. 1 (1998): 5–13.

47. Law, M., S. Baptiste, A. Carwell, M. A. McColl, H. Polotajko, and N. Pollack. *Canadian Occupational Performance Measures.* 2nd ed. Toronto: CAOT Publications ACE, 1994.

48. Lydic, J. S., and C. Steele. (1979). "Assessment of the Quality of Sitting and Gait Patterns in Children with Down Syndrome." *Physical Therapy* 59, no. 12 (1979): 1489–94.

49. Lydic, J. S., M. M. Windsor, M. A. Short, and T. A. Ellis. "Effects of Controlled Rotary Vestibular Stimulation on the Motor Performance of Infants with Down Syndrome." *Physical and Occupational Therapy in Pediatrics* 5, (1985): 93–118.

50. McGuire, Dennis, and Brian Chicoine. *Mental Wellness in Adults with Down Syndrome.* Bethesda, MD: Woodbine House, 2006.

51. Medlen, Joan, ed. "Assistive Technology." *Disability Solutions* 3, no. 2.

52. Meyers, Laura F. "Using Computers to Teach Children with Down Syndrome." In *The Psychobiology of Down Syndrome,* edited by Lynn Nadel. Cambridge, MA: MIT Press, 1988.

53. Miller, L. J., and S. J. Lane. "Toward a Concensus in Terminology in Sensory Integration Theory and Practice: Part 1: Taxonomy of Neurophysiological Processes. *Sensory Integration Special Interest Section Quarterly* 23, no. 1 (2000): 1–4.

54. Murray-Slutsky, Carolyn, and Betty Paris. *Is Sensory or Is It Behavior?* Hollywood, FL: STAR Services, 2004.

55. Naganuma, Gay M. "Early Intervention for Infants with Down Syndrome: Efficacy Research." *Physical and Occupational Therapy in Pediatrics* 71 (1987): 81–92.

56. Niles-Campbell, N., C. Tam, J. Mays, and G. Skidmore. "Understanding the Development of Keyboarding Skills in Children with Fine Motor Difficulties." *OT Now* 10, no. 4 (2008).

57. Nommensen A., and M. Frikkie. "Sensory Integration and Down's Syndrome." *British Journal of Occupational Therapy* 56, no. 12 (1993): 451–54.

58. Oelwein, Patricia Logan. *Teaching Reading to Children with Down Syndrome: A Guide for Parents and Teachers.* Bethesda, MD: Woodbine House, 1995.

59. Olsen, Janice Z. *Handwriting without Tears.* Potomac, MD: Handwriting without Tears, 1997.

60. Perr, A., E. Petra, and C. Burwell. (2000). "An Investigation of the Use and Potential Use of Accessibility Options Built into Computer Operating Systems." New York: New York University, Department of Occupational Therapy, 2000. https://steinhardt.nyu.edu/scmsAdmin/uploads/000/818/PC_Accessibility.pdf

61. PREP Program. *Effective Teaching Strategies for Successful Inclusion: A Focus on Down Syndrome.* Calgary, Alberta: Author, 1999.

62. Rast, M., and S. Harris (1985). "Motor Control in Infants with Down Syndrome." *Developmental Medicine and Child Neurology* 27 (1985): 675–85.

63. Reat, Cristen. "Living Life with Apps." *Down Syndrome News* 35, no. 2 (2012).

64. Reisman, J. E., and B. Hanschu. *Sensory Integration Inventory—Revised for Individuals with Developmental Disabilities: User's Guide.* Hugo, Minnesota: PDP Press, 1992.

65. Russell, D., R. Palisano, S. Walter, P. Rosenbaum, M. Gemus, C. Gowland, B. Galuppi, and M. Lane (1998). "Evaluating Motor Function in Children with Down Syndrome: Validity of the GMFM." *Developmental Medicine and Child Neurology* 41 (1998): 693–701.

66. Sahagian, Sandra D. *A Fine Motor Program for Down Syndrome Preschoolers: A Pilot Study.* Unpublished thesis in partial fulfillment of Masters of Health Science. Hamilton, ON: McMaster University, 1985.

67. Selikowitz, Mark. *Down Syndrome: The Facts.* New York: Oxford Press, 1997.

68. *Sharon, Lois, and Bram's Mother Goose.* Illustrated by Maryann Kovalski. Vancouver, British Columbia: Douglas & McIntyre, 1989.

69. Siegert, J. J., W. P. Cooney, and J. H. Dobyns. "Management of Simple Camptodactyly." *Journal of Hand Surgery* (British Volume) 15B (1990): 181–89.

70. Smith, L., S. Von Tetzchner, B. Michalsen. "The Emergence of Language Skills in Young Children with Down Syndrome." In *The Psychobiology of Down Syndrome,* edited by Lynn Nadel. Cambridge, MA: MIT Press, 1988.

71. Shumway-Cook, A., and M. Woollacott. "Dynamics of Postural Control in the Child with Down Syndrome." *Physical Therapy 33 (9)* (1985): 1315–22.

72. Solomon, Andrew. *Far from the Tree.* Scribner, NY: 2012.

73. Stock Kranowitz, Carol. *The Out-of Sync Child.* New York: Skylight Press, 1998.

74. Thombs, Barry, and David Sugden. "Manual Skills in Down Syndrome Children Ages 6 to 16 Years." *Adapted Physical Activity Quarterly* 8 (1991): 242–54.

75. Uyanik M., G. Bumin, and H. Kayihan. "Comparisons of Different Therapy Approaches in Children with Down Syndrome." *Pediatrics International* 45 (2003): 68–73.

76. Novak Hoffman, M., L. Lusardi Peterson, and D. C. Van Dyke. "Motor and Hand Function." In *Clinical Perspectives in the Management of Down Syndrome,* edited by D. C. Van Dyke, D. J. Lang, F. Heide, S. van Duyne, and M. M. Soucek. New York: Springer-Verlag, 1990.

77. Van Dyke, D. C., P. Mattheis, S. Schoon Eberly, and J. Williams, eds. *Medical and Surgical Care for Children with Down Syndrome.* Bethesda, MD: Woodbine House, 1995.

78. Vermeer, A., and W. E. Davis, eds. "Motor Development in Young Children with Down Syndrome." *Physical and Motor Development in Mental Retardation.* Basel: Karger, 1995.

79. Virji-Babul, N., J. E. V. Lloyd, and G. Van. "Performing Movement Sequences with Knowledge of Results under Different Visual Conditions in Adults with Down Syndrome." *Down Syndrome Research and Practice* 8, no. 3 (2003): 110–14.

80. Vulpe, Shirley German. *Vulpe Assessment Battery.* Toronto: National Institute on Mental Retardation, 1969.

81. Weeks, Daniel J., Romeo Chua, and Digby Elliot, eds. *Perceptual-Motor Behavior in Down Syndrome.* Windsor, Ontario: Human Kinetics, 2000.

82. Williams, Mary Sue, and Sherry Shellenberger. *"How Does Your Engine Run?" A Leader's Guide to the Alert Program for Self-Regulation.* Albuquerque, NM: Therapy Works, 1996

83. Winders, Patricia C. *Gross Motor Skills for Children with Down Syndrome: A Guide for Parents and Professionals.* 2nd ed. Bethesda, MD: Woodbine House, 2014.

84. Wishart, Jennifer. "Motivation and Learning Styles in Young Children with Down Syndrome." *Down Syndrome Research and Practice* 7, no. 2 (2001): 47–51.

85. Wuang, Y. P., and C. Y Su. "Correlations of Sensory Processing and Visual Organization Ability with Participation in School-Aged Children with Down Syndrome." *Research in Developmental Disabilities* 32, no. 6 (2011).

86. Yack, Ellen, Paula Aquilla, and Shirley Sutton. *Building Bridges through Sensory Integration: Therapy for Children with Autism and Other Pervasive Developmental Disorders.* Las Vegas, NV: Sensory Resources, 2002.

87. Zausmer, Elizabeth, and Alice M. Shea. "Motor Development." In *The Young Child with Down Syndrome,* edited by Siegfried Pueschel. New York: Human Sciences Press, 1984.

88. Zausmer, Elizabeth. "Fine Motor Skills and Play." In *A Parent's Guide to Down Syndrome: Toward a Brighter Future,* edited by Siegfried Pueschel. Baltimore: Paul H. Brookes, 1990.

Resources

The resources listed here offer support, information, and/or items that may assist families and children, teens, or adults who have Down syndrome with sensory processing and fine motor skill development, and with general information related to Down syndrome.

Product Sources

ABLEDATA
www.abledata.com
   Information about assistive technology products and rehabilitation equipment.

Ablenet
800-322-0956
www.ablenetinc.com
   Tech access products and tools.

Adaptive Technology Resources
www.adaptivetechnologyresources.com
   Hardware, software, Intellitools, training.

Alert Program for Self-Regulation: How Does Your Engine Run?
Therapy Works Inc.
P.O. Box 95316
Albuquerque, NM 87199
877-897-3478
www.alertprogram.com

App Lists: These websites are examples of many that provide lists of apps for developmental skills:

- Down Syndrome Daily (www.downsyndromedaily.com)
- DSAQ Guide to Apps (http://www.dsaq.org.au/publications/dsaq-guide-to-apps-2nd-edition)
- BridgingApps (www.bridgingapps.org)
- OTs with APPS & Technology (www.otswithapps.com)

Apple Accessibility
800-MY-APPLE
www.apple.com/accessibility
   Information on accessibility options on Mac computers and devices.

Bridges Assistive Technologies
800-353-1107
info@bridges-canada.com
www.bridges-canada.com
   Provides assistive technology products, tech support, and training (Canada).

Different Roads
37 E. 18th St.
New York, NY 10003
800-853-1057
www.difflearn.com
   Products for children with developmental delays and autism, including visual supports, ABA Materials, *Handwriting without Tears* materials, fine motor activities.

Dragonfly: Universal Access Resource
291 Yale Ave.
Winnepeg, MB R3M OL4 Canada
866-559-1086
www.dragonflytoys.com
   Universal access educational video games, software, toys, aids for daily living.

Flaghouse, Inc. (Canada)
235 Yorkland Blvd., Ste. 105
North York, ON M2J 4Y8
800-265-6900
www.flaghouse.ca
   Adapted toys and equipment, Snoezelen equipment, and resources.

Flaghouse, Inc. (U.S.)
601 FlagHouse Dr.
Hasbrouck Heights, NJ 07604
800-793-7900
www.flaghouse.com
Adapted toys and equipment, Snoezelen equipment, and resources.

Fun and Function
P.O. Box 11
Merion Station, PA 19066
800-231-6329
www.funandfunction.com
Focuses on products for sensory regulation and play, as well as calming and focusing.

Handwriting without Tears
806 W. Diamond Ave., Ste. 230
Gaithersburg, MD 20878
301-263-2707
www.hwtears.com
Handwriting without Tears printing and writing program workbook and materials for students of all ages; *Keyboarding without Tears.*

InfoGrip: Assistive Technology Devices and Adaptive Products
1899 E. Main St.
Ventura, CA 93001
800-397-0921
www.infogrip.com
Assistive technology solutions; keyboard, mouse, and monitor adaptations.

Don Johnston, Inc.
26799 W. Commerce Dr.
Volo, IL 60073
800-999-4660
www.donjohnston.com
Intervention resources for reading and writing, including CoWriter and WriteOutLoud.

Mayer-Johnson, Inc.
2100 Wharton St., Ste. 400
Pittsburgh, PA 15203
800-588-4548
www.mayer-johnson.com
    Software (including Boardmaker), hardware, Intellitools, and books.

One Place for Special Needs
www.oneplaceforspecialneeds.com
    Lists a variety of sources for products, as well as online resources such as free social stories.

OTPlan
www.otplan.com
    A search engine that enables you to find activity ideas for skill development in various domains.

The Pencil Grip, Inc.
P.O. Box 3787
Chatsworth, CA 91313
888-736-4747
www.thepencilgrip.com
    Various pencil grips, Gripables cutlery, and other products.

Pocket Full of Therapy
P.O. Box 174
Morganville, NJ 07751
800-PFOT-124
www.pfot.com
    Resources include seat cushions, raised-line paper, scissors; Touch Window (for computer monitor); fine motor activities. Website includes an "idea exchange."

School Specialty
P.O. Box 1529
Appleton, WI 54912-1529
888-388-3224
www.schoolspecialty.com (in the U.S.)
https://store.schoolspecialty.com (in Canada)
    Sells educational products and "special needs" products including the Abilitations brand and many items for sensory needs.

SensorySmarts
info@sensorysmarts.com
www.Sensorysmarts.com
Information provided by the authors of *Raising a Sensory Smart Child* about resources for sensory-based products, toys, and equipment.

SMART Technologies
888-42SMART
Smarttech.com
SMART Boards and other technologies.

Social Stories
www.CarolGraySocialStories.com
Information about Social Stories from the developer of the concept.

Southpaw Enterprises
P.O. Box 1047
Dayton, OH 45401
800-228-1698 (in U.S.); 937-252-6460 (international)
www.southpaw.com
Multisensory equipment and products for developing fine motor and sensory skills.

Tfh Special Needs Toys
4537 Gibsonia Rd.
Gibsonia, PA 15044
800-467-6222
www.specialneedstoys.com
Products for developing personalized sensory environments as well as for working on skills in all developmental areas.

Therapro
225 Arlington St.
Framingham, MA 01702-8723
800-257-5376
www.theraproducts.com
Fine motor, sensory, daily living, therapeutic, and educational products.

Toys "R" Us Toy Guide for Differently Abled Kids
http://www.toysrus.com/shop/index.jsp?categoryId=3261680
The guide categorizes toys that are useful in working on specific skill areas. Available in Spanish. Print copies of the guide are available at Toys R Us stores.

TheraTogs
888-634-0495
www.theratogs.com
    Orthotic garment systems.

Zones of Regulation
Kuypers Consulting
5532 Park Ave.
Minneapolis, MN 55417
312-952-4361
www.zonesofregulation.com
    Book and activities for the Zones of Regulation program, which fosters
self-regulation and emotional control.

Organizations

American Occupational Therapy Association
4720 Montgomery Lane, Ste. 200
Bethesda, MD 20814-3449
301-652-6611
www.aota.org

The Arc of the United States
1825 K Street, NW, Ste. 1200
Washington, DC 20006
800-433-5255; 202-534-3700
www.thearc.org

Autism Society Canada
Box 22017
1670 Heron Road
Ottawa, ON K1V 0W2
866-476-8440; 519-695-5858
info@autismsocietycanada.ca
www.autismsocietycanada.ca

Autism Society of America
4340 East-West Hwy, Ste. 350
Bethesda, MD 20814
800-3-autism (328-8476); 301-657-0881
info@autism-society.org
www.autism-society.org

Canadian Association for Community Living
Kinsmen Building, York University
4700 Keele St.
Toronto, ON M3J 1P3
416-661-9611
inform@cacl.ca
www.cacl.ca

Canadian Association of Occupational Therapists
L'Association Canadienne Des Ergotherapeutes
100-34 Colonnade Rd.
Ottawa, ON K2E 7J6
800-434-2268
www.caot.ca

Canadian Down Syndrome Society
2003 14 Street NW, Ste. 103
Calgary, AB T2M 3N4
800-883-8500
info@cdss.ca
www.cdss.ca

Disability.gov
www.disability.gov

Down Syndrome International
Langdon Down Centre
2A Langdon Park
Teddington, Middlesex
TW11 9PS
United Kingdom
contact@ds-int.org
www.ds-int.org

Down Syndrome Medical Interest Group
www.dsmig-usa.org
www.dsmig.org.uk

Geneva Centre for Autism
112 Merton Street
Toronto, ON M4S 2Z8
416-322-7877
info@autism.net
www.autism.net

Global Down Syndrome Foundation
3300 East First Ave., Ste. 390
Denver, CO 80206
303-321-6277
info@globaldownsyndrome.org
www.globaldownsyndrome.org

LuMind Foundation
(formerly Down Syndrome Research Foundation)
225 Cedar Hill St., Ste. 200
Marlborough, MA 01752
508-630-2177
lumind@lumindfoundation.org
www.lumindfoundation.org

National Down Syndrome Congress
30 Mansell Court, Ste. 108
Roswell, GA 30076
800-232-NDSC
info@ndsccenter.org
www.ndsccenter.org

National Down Syndrome Society
666 Broadway, 8th Floor
New York, NY 10012
800-221-4602
info@ndss.org
www.ndss.org

National Lekotek Center
2001 N. Clybourn Ave., 1st Floor
Chicago, IL 60614
773-528-5766
www.lekotek.org

Index

JUL 2020

JUL 2020

About the Author

Maryanne Bruni's 35-year career as an occupational therapist has included work in clinics, schools, and community settings with infants, preschoolers, and school-aged children. She is now volunteer Board President of West Toronto KEYS to INclusion, a nonprofit charitable organization promoting inclusive opportunities for adults with intellectual disabilities. Her passions include family, music, travel, the outdoors, tennis, hiking, and cycling. She lives with her husband and youngest daughter, who has Down syndrome, in Toronto.